THE ANTI-INFLAMMATORY BOOK FOR WOMEN OVER 40

FEEL YOUR BEST EVERY DAY WITH PROVEN TECHNIQUES TO LOWER INFLAMMATION, BALANCE HORMONES, IMPROVE GUT HEALTH, AND INCREASE ENERGY!

MARUSYA WELLNESS PUBLISHING

"To my friend Nataliya K., You are like a shining star in my life, always there to support and be a wonderful friend. This book is dedicated to you, to express my gratitude for your friendship."

CONTENTS

INTRODUCTION

Getting healthy after 40 isn't just about fixing specific health problems; it's about making changes to your whole life that are good for your mind, body, and spirit. This book is here to tell you that your best years aren't behind you. In fact, you can feel healthy, happy, and brimming with energy every single day if you just take the right steps.

As women step into their 40s and beyond, they start to face different health problems. Changes in hormones, a higher risk of chronic inflammation, changes in metabolism, and evolving gut health needs make the wellness world quite unique at this stage and require special care. This book dives deep into these issues, showing how the complex balance of our bodies shifts over time and giving specific ways to handle these changes.

By this point, being healthy means more than just avoiding being sick. It's about physical vigour, mental clarity, emotional well-being, and spiritual satisfaction. To stay healthy, you've got to take a close look at your diet, habits, and activities to become more mindful. This book looks at how different aspects of health interconnect and shows how a lifestyle low in inflammation can help you improve your overall health.

It is grounded in scientific research, but written in a way that is easy to understand and helpful. Each part was carefully written to guide you in making informed, smart choices about your health by mixing the latest scientific findings with helpful advice. You'll find a mix of recommendations here, from diet suggestions to exercise ideas, ways to deal with stress, and tips for better sleep quality, all specifically for women over 40.

When you start this journey, you promise to care for your body and mind in new ways. As you go through these pages, don't just think of it as reading a book. Think of it as taking the first step on this journey that will change you—a way to live a fuller, healthier, and more fulfilling life. Let's take a step towards this journey together. Our goal is to be healthy and happy and to embrace this newfound knowledge and beauty of being a woman over 40.

You are now on your way to being better and more alive.

UNDERSTANDING INFLAMMATION

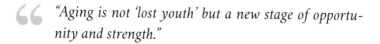

"*Aging is not 'lost youth' but a new stage of opportunity and strength.*"

— *BETTY FRIEDAN*

1.1: DEFINING INFLAMMATION AND ITS ROLE IN THE BODY

Inflammation is a fundamental biological process essential to how the body defends itself. People often think of inflammation as bad, but it's an important immune response that helps the body heal from injuries and fight infections. To fully understand how inflammation affects our health, particularly for women over 40, we need to delve into its nature, how it functions, the different types, its benefits, and what could go wrong if it lasts for a long time.

Firstly, Let's Understand What Inflammation Is

Inflammation is the body's natural reaction to harmful elements like germs, broken cells, or allergens. It's an important part of the immune system, a complex network that keeps us safe from bacteria, viruses, and other dangerous outside invaders, as well as from damaged cells and poisonous substances inside our bodies.

How the Inflammatory Response Works

When our body gets hurt or infected, the body's immune cells are stimulated, releasing different chemicals such as histamines, prostaglandins, and cytokines. These chemicals increase blood flow to the affected area, which causes the usual signs of acute inflammation: redness, heat, swelling, and pain. These extra immune cells and increased blood flow help keep the wound from spreading, which further stops the infection and starts the healing process.

Short-term Vs. Long-term Inflammation

There are two main types of inflammation: acute and chronic. Acute inflammation is a short-term response that has effects that are limited to one area. It usually happens in response to accidents or diseases. It usually goes away very quickly in a few days after it begins. On the other hand, chronic inflammation lasts for a long time and is generally less severe but can last for months or even years. It can happen because of long-lasting infections, allergens, autoimmune diseases, or chronic illnesses.

The Inflammation Sword with Two Edges

Acute inflammation is actually your body's way of protecting and healing itself, but on the flip side, chronic inflammation can lead to a whole bunch of health issues. Think heart disease, arthritis, diabetes, cancer, and neurological diseases —these are all linked to long-lasting inflammation that ends up damaging tissues. When the inflammatory response lasts for a long time, or the body can't eliminate the cause of inflammation, it shifts from being an acute inflammation to a chronic one.

Women Over 40 With Inflammation

Now, for women over 40, inflammation is especially important. Hormonal changes, especially around menopause, can really affect the body's inflammation reaction. Less estrogen in the body can make chronic inflammatory diseases worse because estrogen reduces inflammation. With this hormonal shift, women are at a higher risk of developing inflammation-linked diseases, such as osteoporosis, heart disease, and various inflammatory disorders.

How to Find and Treat Chronic Inflammation

A lot of the time, chronic inflammation doesn't show up as clearly as acute inflammation. This makes it more sneakier and harder to spot. It can show up as tiredness, joint pain, skin problems, stomach problems, and weight gain. Tackling chronic inflammation isn't a one-size-fits-all approach. Instead, it requires a multifaceted approach that includes changing your diet to include more anti-inflammatory foods, regular exercise, learning how to deal with stress, and, sometimes, taking medicine.

What You Eat Can Cause Inflammation

A big part of controlling inflammation comes down to what's on your plate. Some foods, like those high in vitamins, omega-3 fatty acids, and antioxidants, can help lower inflammation. Some are whole grains, nuts, fruits and veggies, and fatty fish. On the flip side, processed foods, a sugar spree, and going overboard with red meat and not-so-great fats can worsen inflammation.

What role does medical intervention play?

Chronic inflammation may sometimes need medical help to be managed. This can include taking anti-inflammatory drugs, going through hormone replacement therapy (for women who have gone through menopause), and getting better from other health problems that might be causing the chronic inflammation.

Final Thoughts

Inflammation is a very important biological reaction that has many bodily functions. It's very important to understand the balance between how it can help in emergencies and how it can hurt over time, particularly for women over 40. You can successfully control inflammation and improve your health and well-being by spotting the signs of chronic inflammation and taking steps such as making changes to your food and lifestyle and getting medical help. This insight gives you the power to take charge of your health, which is especially important for women in their 40s and older who face special problems.

1.2: THE SPECIFIC IMPACT OF INFLAMMATION ON WOMEN'S HEALTH POST-40

When the immune system responds to inflammation, it has a unique impact on women's health, particularly after hitting the 40-year mark. During this time, which is often marked by perimenopause and menopause, hormones change in ways that have a big effect on how women's bodies respond to inflammation. You need to understand this link to keep your health in good shape and avoid health risks at this point in your life.

Changes in Hormones and Inflammation

Women's estrogen levels drop as they age, especially after age 40. Estrogen can reduce inflammation, help keep the immune system in check, and keep the skin and blood vessels healthy. However, for women going through peri-menopause or menopause, the loss of estrogen can make their bodies more inflamed. This increased inflammation can worsen diseases and raise the risk of developing new ones.

A Higher Chance of Getting Chronic Diseases

After age 40, inflammation levels tend to rise, making you more likely to develop chronic illnesses. Some of these are:

- **Cardiovascular Disease**: Women over 40 are more likely to get heart disease. This is partly because they have more inflammation, which can cause a build-up of artery plaque and high blood pressure.
- **Osteoporosis:** Inflammation can speed up bone loss, raising osteoporosis risk. This is a problem that

many women after menopause have because their estrogen levels have dropped.

- **Type 2 Diabetes:** Long-term inflammation can make insulin less effective, increasing the risk of type 2 diabetes.
- **Autoimmune Diseases**: Women are more likely than men to get autoimmune diseases, and people over 40 are more likely to get rheumatoid arthritis and lupus, both of which involve inflammation.

Inflammation Linked to Menopause

As a woman goes through menopause, she might find herself dealing with more inflammation. Having hot flashes and night sweats is not only uncomfortable, but it can also be a sign of an inflammatory reaction. Adipose tissue (fat) is known to release pro-inflammatory cytokines, which can make inflammation even worse. During this time, weight gain is pretty common because of those hormonal changes.

The Effect on Mental Health

Inflammation isn't just a physical issue after age 40. It can seriously affect mental health, too. The rollercoaster of emotions—like mood swings, sadness, and anxiety—that often accompanies the perimenopausal period might have more to do with inflammation than we thought. More and more evidence suggests that these mental health problems are linked to inflammation. Managing inflammation may help keep mental health in good shape.

Skin and Responses to Inflammation

Since the skin is the biggest organ, it is also affected by changes in inflammation. A drop in estrogen levels means less collagen production and reduced skin elasticity, making the skin more prone to inflammation, dryness, and the visible signs of aging.

Digestive Health and Adverse Events

When a woman turns 40, her gut health often changes. Irritable bowel syndrome (IBS) and gastric reflux disease (GERD) are two conditions where inflammation plays a big role. The gut flora, which changes as people age, is crucial for controlling the body's reaction to inflammation.

The Inflammatory Response to Stress

As people age, their ability to deal with worry may decrease, strengthening their inflammation reaction. It is known that long-term worry can raise cortisol levels, which can then make inflammation worse. For women over 40, this is especially important because they often have to balance many things, like work, family, and their own health.

Lifestyle Factors That Affect Inflammation

What you eat, how much you move, and the quality of your sleep, among other things, greatly impact how well they control inflammation. To keep inflammation under control, you need to eat many anti-inflammatory foods, stay active, and get enough sleep. It's also important to stop smoking and avoid alcohol

Ways to Deal with Inflammation

When it comes to food, a diet full of fruits, veggies, whole grains, and omega-3 fatty acids can help lower inflammation.

- **Exercise**: Regular physical activity, from running routines to muscle training, can decrease levels of inflammatory markers.
- **Stress Management**: Practices like yoga, meditation, and mindfulness can be powerful tools for dealing with stress and reducing inflammation.
- **Medical Care**: For some women, consider hormone replacement therapy (HRT) with the help of a doctor because it can help lessen some of the inflammatory effects of menopause.

Final Thoughts

In conclusion, inflammation significantly impacts the health of women over 40, influencing their physical and mental well-being as well as their overall quality of life. Understanding these changes is important for developing effective ways to deal with the health risks of higher inflammation. By changing their lifestyles and seeing a doctor when needed, women can handle these changes more easily and enjoy a healthier, more peaceful life after 40.

1.3: IDENTIFYING COMMON INFLAMMATORY TRIGGERS IN DAILY LIFE

When everyday things cause inflammation regularly, it can become a problem. Inflammation is a normal immune response to damage or illness. Understanding and naming these causes is important for controlling and avoiding inflammation you don't want, particularly for people over 40 who might be more susceptible. This in-depth look at the various day-to-day factors that can cause inflammation and how they can be lessened is an in-depth analysis of the topic.

What You Eat and How Healthy It is

Diet is arguably the most important daily cause of inflammation. Certain foods are known to make the body react with inflammation:

- **Processed and Refined Foods**: Fast food, baked goods, and processed snacks high in refined sugars and trans fats can cause these reactions.
- **Red and processed meats:** These meats have a lot of advanced glycation end products (AGEs), which cause inflammation and heavy fats.
- **Dairy Products**: Some people, especially those who are lactose intolerant or sensitive to dairy, can get inflammation from consuming dairy products.

Being Overweight and Having Body Fat

Visceral fat around the belly is extra body fat that does more than store calories—it's also an active endocrine system that causes inflammation by releasing cytokines. This can cause the body to have low-level inflammation all the time.

They need to move around more.

Chronic diseases linked to inflammation, like heart disease and type 2 diabetes, can get worse if you don't do enough physical exercise daily. On the other hand, exercise is known to reduce inflammation in the body.

Long-Term Stress

The adrenal glands produce the hormone cortisol when you're dealing with a lot of stress. First, cortisol reduces inflammation. However, long-term stress and cortisol release can worsen the body's ability to regulate inflammation, leading to chronic inflammation.

Toxins in the Environment

Pollution, cigarette smoke, and industrial chemicals are everyday outdoor toxins that can cause inflammatory reactions. Cells can be damaged by these toxins, which can lead to inflammation.

I am not getting enough sleep.

Skimping on sleep, both in quantity and quality, can mess up the body's normal reactions to inflammation. Chronic lack of sleep is linked to higher amounts of chemicals that cause inflammation.

Gut Health and an Imbalance of Microbiota

The bacteria present in your gut are very important for regulating your immune system. If you don't eat well or take antibiotics, your gut bacteria can become out of balance. This can cause your intestinal permeability to rise, which further leads to bacteria and toxins entering your system, causing inflammation.

Long-term Illnesses and Infections

Even minor diseases that last for a long time can keep the immune system on high alert, which can cause inflammation to last for a long time. This is very clear in conditions like gum disease.

Getting Older

Our bodies' natural ability to control the inflammatory reaction can weaken as we age, raising the risk of chronic inflammation. This is especially important for people over 40.

Allergies and Disorders of the Nervous System

Some people can have inflammation reactions to common allergens like pollen, pet hair, and some foods. Autoimmune diseases, in which the body's immune system fights its own organs, are also naturally inflammatory.

Plans to Reduce Inflammatory Triggers

- **Changing your diet** to include more fruits, veggies, whole grains, lean protein, and healthy fats can help lower inflammation.
- **Regular Physical Activity**: A mix of aerobic and strength training routines can help reduce inflammation.
- **Stress Management Techniques**: Yoga, meditation, and awareness are some practices that can help you deal with stress and the inflammation that comes with it.

- **Improving Sleep Hygiene**: Making a normal sleep routine and making your bedroom a good place to sleep can help lower inflammation.
- **Reducing Exposure to Environmental Toxins**: Not smoking or drinking and reducing exposure to pollution are all examples that can make a lot of difference.
- **Maintaining Gut Health:** A diet high in fiber, probiotics, and prebiotics can help keep gut bacteria balanced.
- **Taking care of long-term illnesses:** Regular checkups and medicines for diabetes, obesity, and heart disease can help lower inflammation.
- **Hydration and Healthy Lifestyle Choices**: Staying hydrated and healthy can also help reduce inflammation.

Final Thoughts

To sum up, your daily habits and choices have a big impact on inflammation, which can be fixed by changing how you live. People, especially those over the age of 40, can significantly lower their risk of chronic inflammation and the health problems that come with it by identifying and addressing these triggers. This proactive approach includes changing your food, exercising more, dealing with stress, and being more aware of your surroundings. It will help you live a better, more balanced life.

Here is a table summarizing the common inflammatory triggers in daily life and strategies to mitigate them:

Inflammatory Triggers	Strategies to Mitigate
Diet and Nutritional Factors	- Adopt an anti-inflammatory diet with fruits, vegetables, whole grains, and lean protein. Avoid processed, refined foods, excessive red meat, and high sugar intake.
Obesity and Body Fat	- Manage weight through a balanced diet and regular exercise.
Physical Inactivity	- Incorporate regular physical activity, including both aerobic and resistance exercises.
Chronic Stress	- Engage in stress management techniques such as yoga, meditation, and mindfulness.
Environmental Toxins	- Minimize exposure to pollutants, avoid smoking, and alcohol consumption.
Poor Sleep Habits	- Improve sleep hygiene by establishing a regular sleep schedule and creating a sleep-friendly environment.
Gut Health and Microbiota Imbalance	- Balance gut bacteria with probiotics, prebiotics, and a fiber-rich diet.
Chronic Infections and Illnesses	- Regular medical check-ups and managing existing health conditions effectively.

Aging	- Engage in healthy lifestyle choices, regular exercise, and a balanced diet to mitigate natural inflammatory responses due to aging.
Allergies and Autoimmune Disorders	- Identify and manage allergies with appropriate treatments; monitor and treat autoimmune disorders under medical guidance.
Hydration and Lifestyle Choices	- Ensure adequate hydration and overall healthy lifestyle choices.

This table provides a concise overview of how daily lifestyle factors can trigger inflammation and the practical steps one can take to reduce or manage these triggers, especially for individuals over 40 years of age.

1.4: THE RELATIONSHIP BETWEEN CHRONIC INFLAMMATION AND DISEASES

Chronic inflammation, an inflammatory reaction lasting for a long time, is a big part of how many illnesses start and worsen. While acute inflammation is good for you and important for healing, ongoing inflammation can be bad for your health. Here, we look more deeply into the complex relationship between long-term inflammation and several illnesses, mainly those affecting people over 40.

Learn about chronic inflammation.

Inflammatory markers are made slowly and continuously in people with chronic inflammation. It can happen because of acute inflammation that isn't treated, infections that won't go away, autoimmune reactions, or long-term exposure to irritants like pollution or poor eating habits. Unlike acute inflammation, which goes away once the body heals, chronic inflammation lingers, potentially damaging tissues and systems over time, often without any obvious symptoms.

Long-term Inflammation and Cardiovascular Diseases

Heart disease, stroke, and other cardiovascular illnesses (CVD) are all linked to chronic inflammation. In people with CVD, inflammatory markers like C-reactive protein (CRP) are often higher. This inflammation process can worsen atherosclerosis, a condition in which fatty deposits build up on the walls of arteries and make them thicker. Plaques, these deposits, can break apart and form blood clots that can block blood flow or break off and go to other parts of the body, where they could cause a heart attack or stroke.

What Effects It Has on Metabolic Disorders

An important part of how metabolic diseases like type 2 diabetes and obesity start is chronic inflammation. Too much fatty tissue makes pro-inflammatory molecules that worsen insulin resistance, a sign of type 2 diabetes. People who are overweight or fat have a chronic inflammation state that makes diabetes worse and makes it harder to control.

Diseases That Cause Long-term Inflammation

An inflammatory disease like rheumatoid arthritis, a gut disease like Crohn's disease, ulcerative colitis, or eczema happens naturally. When someone has these diseases, their immune system accidentally hits good tissues, leading to ongoing inflammation and damage to the tissues.

Cancer and Long-term Inflammation

Chronic inflammation has been found to play a big role in the growth and spread of many types of cancer. Inflammation that doesn't go away can damage DNA and encourage abnormalities that can lead to cancer. People with inflammatory conditions, such as chronic hepatitis, may be more likely to get liver cancer. People with inflammatory gut diseases are also more likely to get colon cancer.

Diseases of the Nervous System

There is more and more proof that brain diseases like Alzheimer's, Parkinson's, and multiple sclerosis are linked to chronic inflammation. Neurodegenerative diseases are linked to inflammatory processes that can damage neurons and play a role in how they progress.

Diseases of the Lungs

Asthma and chronic obstructive pulmonary disease (COPD) are two lung diseases in which long-term inflammation is very important. In these cases, inflammation makes breathing hard because it narrows the airways, making breathing difficult and significantly impacting quality of life.

The Effect on Age (Inflammation)

Inflammaging is the term for the idea that chronic inflammation can speed up the aging process. Older individuals often experience low-level systemic inflammation, which is linked to age-related diseases such as arthritis, osteoporosis, and cognitive decline.

The Part Lifestyle and Environment Play

Your lifestyle choices, including diet, physical activity, stress management, and exposure to environmental toxins, have a major impact on chronic inflammation. Eating lots of processed foods, sugars, and bad fats can worsen inflammation, whereas doing regular exercise and learning how to deal with stress can help reduce it.

Ways to Deal with Long-Term Inflammation

Taking care of chronic inflammation requires more than one step:

Eat a diet low in inflammation-causing substances and high in carbohydrates, omega-3 fatty acids, and vitamins.

- **Exercise**: It is known that regular exercise can lower inflammation markers.
- **Managing your weight**: Keeping a healthy weight can make chronic inflammation easier.
- **Reduction of stress**: Mindfulness, meditation, and yoga are all techniques that can help reduce inflammation caused by stress.
- **Medical Management**: You may need anti-inflammatory drugs or disease-modifying agents to control chronic inflammation.

Final Thoughts

In the end, prolonged inflammation is a major cause of the start and spread of many illnesses, particularly in people over 40. It impacts various organ systems and can cause various health problems, from metabolic illnesses to neurological diseases. Understanding how chronic inflammation affects disease processes is important for developing ways to prevent and manage these conditions effectively. The effects of chronic inflammation can be greatly reduced by changing one's lifestyle and getting the right medical care. This can pave the way for healthier and longer lives.

1.5: STRATEGIES FOR RECOGNIZING AND DOCUMENTING INFLAMMATORY RESPONSES

Recognizing and documenting inflammatory reactions is key to understanding and dealing with possible health problems, especially as we grow older. Chronic inflammation can be a hidden cause of many diseases, so it's important to figure out what it is for effective health management. This in-depth section outlines various ways to spot signs of inflammation and how you can properly record them for better health results. This is particularly important for people over 40, who are more likely to have chronic inflammation.

Knowing the Signs of Inflammation

There are many obvious and less obvious ways that inflammation can show up. Recognizing these signs is the first crucial step that needs to be taken to deal with these possible problems:

- **Physical Symptoms**: Redness, swelling, heat, and pain in certain places are common signs. However, prolonged inflammation can manifest as tiredness, general pain, stomach problems, or weight changes, which you can't explain.

- **Responses that are "acute" vs. "chronic":** Tell the difference between acute inflammation, a normal part of the healing process, and chronic inflammation, which is less obvious and lasts longer. It's harder to spot chronic inflammation because it doesn't always have strong signs of acute inflammation.

Self-Monitoring and Writing in a Journal

Keeping a health log is one of the best ways to spot and record inflammation. Here's how you can go about it:

- **Daily Symptom Tracking**: Write down your symptoms everyday, no matter how unimportant they seem. Write down any times you feel pain, stiffness, swelling, or other unusual feelings.
- **Diet and Lifestyle Correlation**: Write down what you eat and how you live. Some foods or hobbies may be linked to the start or improvement of symptoms.
- **Emotional and Mental Health**: Chronic inflammation can affect your mental health. Keep track of changes in your mood, stress, and mental health issues.

Making Use of Health Apps and Tech

Use technology to make your paperwork more accurate. Several health apps let you keep track of your symptoms, food, exercise, and even your mental health, giving you a full picture of your health.

Regular Check-ups With a Doctor and Biomarker Testing

Regular check-ups with your doctor can help you find signs of inflammation. Talk to your doctor about tests that measure markers, such as C-reactive protein (CRP) and Erythrocyte Sedimentation Rate (ESR), among other things, to pinpoint triggers of Inflammatory Responses.

To manage and understand what triggers your inflammatory responses, it's important to consider various factors. Common culprits include certain foods, stress, external factors, and not getting enough sleep. By keeping track of when symptoms get worse, these causes can be found more easily.

Medical Imaging and Lab Tests

In some cases, imaging studies and lab tests may be needed to understand the level and effects of inflammation fully. These include blood tests, MRIs, and X-rays, especially if you've pain in the joints.

Evaluation of Your Lifestyle

Look at the parts of your body that might cause inflammation:

- **Diet Analysis:** Eating a lot of processed foods, sugars, and unhealthy fats can ramp up inflammation. On the other hand, a diet low in inflammation can help ease symptoms.
- **Physical Activity**: Not working out can worsen inflammation, but exercising regularly can prevent it.
- **Worry and Sleep:** Long-term worry and bad sleep habits are known to make inflammation worse.

Talking to Trained Medical Professionals

It is very important to have regular appointments with medical workers. They can advise you on how to deal with your problems and, if necessary, suggest more tests or treatments.

Learning More About Inflammation

Understanding how inflammation works biologically and its effects can help us recognize and take care of it. Use reputable sites to learn more or ask healthcare professionals for help.

Community and Help Groups

Joining online or community groups can be a great way to learn how others manage and document their inflammatory responses. Sharing your stories can help you in the real world and make you feel better emotionally.

How the Body Reacts to Medicines and Supplements

Keeping track of how your body reacts to anti-inflammatory drugs, vitamins, or changes in food can help you figure out what's most effective for you.

Monitoring for a Long Time

Chronic inflammation requires long-term tracking. Keeping track of and going over symptoms over time can help you see patterns and see which control methods are most effective.

Final Thoughts

In conclusion, noticing and writing down inflammatory reactions is a process that includes self-monitoring, talking to a doctor, evaluating your lifestyle, and learning more. People over 40 should pay close attention to the minor, subtle signs of chronic inflammation and maintain detailed health records. This can help them manage their health and stop inflammation-related diseases from worsening. Using technology in the right way and talking to healthcare workers can help enhance these strategies, ultimately leading to improved health results.

HORMONAL HARMONY

"THE GROUNDWORK OF ALL HAPPINESS IS HEALTH." - LEIGH HUNT

2.1: NAVIGATING THE LANDSCAPE OF HORMONAL CHANGES AFTER 40

After hitting the age of 40, a big change happens in your life, especially for women, because it's often the beginning of perimenopause—the phase leading up to menopause. Hormones change during this time and affect your physical, social, and emotional health. You need to understand and deal with these changes to maintain your health and quality of life. In this chapter, we delve deeply into the changes in hormones after age 40, their impacts, and ways to handle them well.

Know How Hormones Change After Age 40

As women approach menopause, the slow drop in estrogen and progesterone levels is the most important change for most after age 40. These hormones are important for controlling periods, keeping your bones strong, and affecting your mood and energy levels. When these hormones drop, it can lead to various symptoms and health changes.

Symptoms and Effects That Are Common

- **Irregular Periods**: Periods may become less regular, heavier, lighter, or farther apart.
- **When you have hot flashes** or night sweats, you feel very warm suddenly and usually sweat a lot, particularly at night.
- **Mood Swings and Emotional Changes:** Mood swings, anger, and feelings of depression or anxiety can be caused by hormone levels that change.
- **Sleep Disturbances:** Hormonal changes and night sweats can cause insomnia or disrupt sleep patterns.
- **Changes in the vaginal and urine tract:** Lower estrogen levels can make the vaginal area dry, make sex more painful, and raise the risk of urinary tract infections.
- **Less dense bones:** Lower estrogen levels can cause bones to become less dense, raising the risk of osteoporosis.
- **Changes in Weight and Metabolism:** You might notice your metabolism slowing down, leading to weight gain, particularly around your midsection.

Being Aware of How Different Experiences Are

Remembering that hormonal changes after age 40 affect women differently is important. Some people may have very bad symptoms, while others may only feel slight pain. These things can happen depending on your genes, your lifestyle habits, your overall health, and your past sexual history.

Different Ways to Deal With Symptoms

- **Hormone Replacement Therapy (HRT):** HRT can help some women with their menopause symptoms. However, talking to a healthcare worker about the pros and cons is important.
- **Diet and Nutrition**: A healthy, well-balanced diet high in phytoestrogens, calcium, and vitamin D can help control symptoms and improve general health. Cutting back on coffee, alcohol, and spicy foods can ease hot flashes.
- **Regular Exercise**: Working out can help you lose weight, feel better, build stronger bones, and improve your overall health.
- **Stress Management Techniques**: Mindfulness, yoga, and meditation are some practices that can help you deal with mood swings and mental pain.
- **Sleep hygiene:** Creating a comfortable sleep setting, sticking to a normal sleep schedule, and refraining from using drugs before bed can all help you sleep better.
- **Vaginal moisturizers** and lubricants can help you with dryness and pain in the vaginal area during sex.

Keeping an Eye on Bone Health

To avoid osteoporosis, it is important to get regular bone density tests and eat a lot of calcium and vitamin D. Weight-bearing workouts are also good for your bones.

Taking Care of Mental Health

It's important to put mental health first, given the increased risk of mood swings and sadness. Help can be found in counselling or therapy; for some people, medication may be necessary.

Getting Regular Health Checks

After age 40, it's more important to get regular checkups, such as mammograms, pelvic exams, and cholesterol checks, to monitor for health problems that can occur because of hormone changes.

Looking for Help

Support groups, whether in person or online, can offer comfort and useful help from others who are experiencing similar challenges.

Learning on Your Own and Talking to Others

It's important to encourage yourself to learn about the changes that happen after age 40. During this time, it's important to keep lines of communication open with health-care workers, partners, and support networks.

Thinking About Alternative Treatments

Acupuncture, plant pills, and homoeopathy are unusual treatments that help some women. However, talking to medical professionals before beginning any new treatment is important.

Final Thoughts

Finally, figuring out how to deal with hormonal changes after 40 requires a well-rounded approach involving medical, social, and mental strategies. With some careful planning and a clear understanding of how these changes impact each of us individually, the shift can go more smoothly during this time. Women can handle the difficulties and look forward to this stage of life with strength and confidence by making healthy living choices, getting the right medical care, and having a solid support network.

2.2: EXPLORING THE CONNECTION BETWEEN HORMONES AND INFLAMMATION

Knowing how the body reacts to different internal and external factors requires in-depth knowledge and understanding of the complex relationship between hormones and inflammation. Many people, especially those over 40, are more likely to experience hormonal changes, so this relationship is especially important because it affects their overall health and happiness. This section looks at how this link works, its effects, and what it means for managing our health more broadly.

The Role of Hormones and the Inflammatory Response

Hormones are important chemical messengers for controlling many bodily functions, such as the immune system and inflammation. Progesterone, estrogen, testosterone, and cortisol are some of the most important hormones that directly and indirectly affect inflammation.

Estrogen and Pain

Inflammation and estrogen, in particular, have a complex relationship. It can either reduce inflammation or increase it, depending on how much of it is present and which estrogen receptors are in different organs. During the childbearing years, estrogen tends to reduce inflammation, which helps keep the immune system in balance. However, as estrogen levels drop with menopause, the risk of chronic inflammatory diseases can increase.

Progesterone, Testosterone, and Swelling

Progesterone also affects inflammation and the immune system. It generally reduces inflammation and supports the body's defences during pregnancy. As the primary hormone in men, testosterone tries to stop the immune system from reacting too strongly, which makes it anti-inflammatory.

Keeping Cortisol and Inflammation in Check

In response to stress, your body releases cortisol, a steroid hormone that reduces inflammation by slowing down your defence system. But here's the catch: constant stress that causes cortisol to stay in the body for a long time can mess up this control function, making the body more susceptible to inflammation.

Hormones and Autoimmune Diseases

Changes in hormones can cause many autoimmune illnesses, which happen when the body's immune system attacks its tissues by accident. Sex hormones may affect how well the immune system works, since these diseases are more common in women. Depending on the disease and the person, changes in hormone levels can either make inflammatory reactions worse or better.

Hormones, Aging, and Inflammation

As we get older, hormonal changes can lead to "inflammaging," a condition characterized by persistent, low-grade inflammation, particularly in women going through menopause. This is connected to age-related diseases such as osteoporosis, heart disease, and type 2 diabetes.

Hormonal Birth Control and Hormone Replacement Therapy

Hormonal birth control and hormone replacement therapy (HRT) can significantly change the inflammation reaction. While they may regulate hormone levels and reduce inflammation for some, they could potentially increase inflammation in others.

Lifestyle Choices and Their Impact on Hormones and Inflammation

Hormone balance and inflammation levels can be affected by what you eat, how much you exercise, how stressed you are, and how well you sleep. For example, a diet high in processed foods and sugars can reduce hormone balance and worsen inflammation. On the other hand, regular exercise and managing stress effectively can help hormones work better and decrease inflammatory markers.

Ways to Keep Hormones in Check and Control Inflammation

- **Changes to your diet:** Eating anti-inflammatory foods like phytoestrogens, omega-3 fatty acids, and vitamins can help balance your hormones and reduce inflammation.
- **Regular exercise:** Staying active can positively influence your hormone levels and has been linked to reduced inflammation markers.
- **Stress Management**: Techniques like yoga, meditation, and mindfulness can help regulate hormones and reduce inflammation caused by stress.
- **Adequate Sleep**: Ensuring you get enough quality sleep is important for keeping your hormones in check and lowering inflammation.
- **Medical Treatments:** In some cases, medical treatments such as hormone replacement therapy (HRT) or pain management medications might be necessary. These should be carefully considered with the help of medical experts.

Regular Health Check-ups

Regular check-ups with your doctor can help you identify and address hormonal imbalances or heightened inflammation early on by keeping an eye on your hormone levels and inflammatory markers.

Final Thoughts

To sum up, the relationship between hormones and inflammation is both dynamic and intricate, significantly impacting health, particularly as we age. Understanding this connection is important for developing effective ways to maintain hormonal balance and manage inflammation. People can deal with these changes and lessen their effects on their health and quality of life by changing their lifestyle, eating, dealing with stress, and getting medical advice.

2.3: TECHNIQUES FOR ACHIEVING HORMONAL BALANCE NATURALLY

Maintaining your hormones is essential for your overall health and well-being, especially as you go through the changes that come with aging. Hormonal shifts can cause a wide range of health problems, from changes in mood and weight gain to more dangerous conditions like diabetes and heart disease. Although hormonal changes are a natural part of aging, particularly after 40, there are natural remedies and lifestyle changes that can help you restore or maintain balance. Here, we look at useful, all-natural ways for men and women to achieve hormonal balance.

Changes to Your Diet for Better Hormone Health

Adopting an anti-inflammatory diet rich in foods that promote hormonal balance is key. Eating a lot of fruits, veggies, whole grains, lean meats, and healthy fats like Omega-3-rich fish, bananas, and nuts will help you in the long run.

- **Phytoestrogens**: Flaxseeds, soy, and some beans are all good for you because they contain phytoestrogens, which act like estrogen and can be particularly helpful for women experiencing menopause.
- **Limit processed foods and sugar:** Cutting back on processed foods, artificial carbs, and sweets can help balance hormones and reduce inflammation.
- **Adequate Protein Intake**: Eating enough protein at each meal can give you important amino acids that help your body produce and regulate hormones.

Doing Regular Physical Activity

- **Exercise Regularly**: Regular exercise, such as running and strength training, can significantly influence hormone levels by lowering insulin levels and making the body more sensitive to this hormone.
- **Exercises that lower stress:** Yoga and Pilates are not only great for your body but also help lower stress, which is important for maintaining hormonal balance.

Dealing With Stress

- **Awareness and relaxation techniques:** Practices such as meditation, deep breathing exercises, and mindfulness can effectively lower cortisol levels. Cortisol is a stress hormone that can become unbalanced during periods of stress.

- **Adequate Sleep**: Making sleep a priority and maintaining a regular sleep schedule can help control the production of important hormones like insulin, growth hormone, and cortisol.

Herbs and Supplements That Are Natural

- **Adaptogens**: These are natural substances found in plants like Ashwagandha, Rhodiola, and holy basil that help the body fight and manage stress reactions while promoting hormonal balance.
- **Vitamin and Mineral Supplements**: Make sure you get enough vitamins and minerals, such as zinc, magnesium, vitamin D, and B vitamins, since they help your hormones stay healthy. You can get these from food or through vitamin supplements.

Good Gut Health

- **Probiotics and prebiotics**: Good gut bacteria are necessary for hormonal balance. To keep your gut healthy, eat foods high in probiotics, like yogurt, kefir, and fermented veggies, and foods high in prebiotics, like garlic, onions, and bananas.
- **Please do not use too many antibiotics**: Antibiotics are sometimes important, but using them too much can disrupt your gut bacteria, leading to hormonal imbalance.

Keeping Endocrine Disruptors in Check

- **Avoid chemicals:** Chemicals found in plastics, personal care products, and household cleaners can interfere with your hormones. Choose green or organic items whenever you can.

Drinking Water

- **Stay Hydrated:** Getting enough water is important for your health and can help keep your hormones balanced.

Regular Check-ups With a Doctor

- **Check Hormone Levels**: Regularly seeing a doctor for check-ups can help you monitor your hormone levels and will also help you in addressing problems early on. Talking about symptoms and possible alternative treatments can be helpful.

Final Thoughts

To sum up, naturally balancing your hormones requires changing your diet, working out regularly, dealing with stress, getting enough sleep, and using supplements and natural herbs smartly. Even though these methods can be very helpful, it's still important to look at hormonal health as a whole and get specific advice from a doctor, especially if you have serious hormonal issues or health concerns.

Here is a table summarizing the natural techniques for achieving hormonal balance:

Technique	Description and Benefits
Nutritional Adjustments	- Anti-inflammatory diet with fruits, vegetables, lean proteins, whole grains, and healthy fats. Include phytoestrogens and limit processed foods and sugars. Adequate protein intake is crucial.
Regular Physical Activity	- Engage in both aerobic and strength training exercises. Stress-reducing exercises like yoga and Pilates can also be beneficial.
Stress Management	- Practices like meditation, deep breathing, and mindfulness help reduce cortisol levels. Prioritize sleep for hormonal regulation.
Natural Supplements and Herbs	- Use adaptogens like Ashwagandha and Rhodiola. Ensure intake of essential vitamins and minerals, such as Vitamin D, B vitamins, magnesium, and zinc.
Gut Health	- Consume probiotic-rich foods and prebiotics to support a healthy gut microbiome. Avoid overuse of antibiotics.
Limiting Endocrine Disruptors	- Reduce exposure to chemicals in plastics, personal care products, and cleaners that can disrupt hormonal balance. Choose natural or organic products.

Hydration	- Maintain adequate hydration, as it is vital for overall health and hormonal balance.
Regular Health Check-ups	- Monitor hormone levels through regular check-ups with a healthcare provider to identify imbalances and discuss natural remedies.

This table provides a comprehensive overview of the various natural methods available to achieve and maintain hormonal balance, particularly useful for individuals over the age of 40 experiencing hormonal changes.

2.4: UNDERSTANDING THE ROLE OF MENOPAUSE IN HORMONAL HEALTH

When a woman hits menopause, her periods stop. This big event in her life usually happens in her late 40s or early 50s. But it's more than just a shift in her reproductive system. It's also a major chemical change that impacts many health areas. The ovaries stop making as much estrogen and progesterone during this time, which marks the end of a woman's normal fertile years. To deal with the effects of menopause on hormone health, you need to understand the role of menopause first.

The Changes That Come With Menopause

The phase leading up to menopause is called perimenopause, and it can stretch over several years. During this time, women's hormone levels, especially estrogen levels, change, which can lead to a variety of symptoms. Menopause is officially identified when a woman hasn't had her period for 12 months in a row.

The Changes in Hormones That Happen During Menopause

Less estrogen and progesterone in the body is the most important change during menopause. Estrogen controls monthly cycles and does other things in the body, like keeping your bones strong, skin flexible, and the heart healthy. A decline in estrogen levels has a significant impact on these areas.

Signs and Symptoms of Menopause

- **Vasomotor Symptoms:** Night sweats and hot flashes are the most common vasomotor symptoms, affecting more than 75% of women going through menopause.
- **Emotional Well-being:** Mood swings, worry, sadness, and restlessness are some of the psychological symptoms that can happen when hormones change.
- **Vaginal and Urinary Changes**: Less estrogen can make the vaginal area dry, making it painful to urinate, and also raising the risk of getting a UTI.
- **Sleep Disturbances:** People have trouble sleeping and experience insomnia, often worsened by night sweats.
- **Changes in the body:** Women may notice changes in how their weight is distributed, their skin structure, and the health of their hair.

Effects on Health in the Long Term

When it comes to osteoporosis, estrogen is very important for bone health. Lower levels increase the risk of osteoporosis and broken bones.

- **Cardiovascular Health**: Estrogen helps protect the heart. With less estrogen, the risk of heart disease goes up.
- **Cognitive Changes**: More and more studies are looking into the link between a drop in estrogen and cognitive processes, such as remembering or memory.

Ways to Deal with the Symptoms of Menopause

- **Lifestyle changes,** like eating a healthy diet high in calcium and vitamin D, doing regular weight-bearing exercise, and giving up smoking, can significantly reduce some of the health risks of menopause.
- **Hormone Replacement Therapy (HRT):** HRT can help some women with menopause symptoms and lower their risk of getting osteoporosis. However, talking to a healthcare worker about the pros and cons is important.
- **Different Therapies:** Phytoestrogens, plant pills, and acupuncture are some of the different methods that have helped some women.
- **Mental Health Support**: Talking to a counsellor or therapist can help you deal better with your mental health issues, which might be a result of menopause.

Why Health Screenings Are Important

Women who have gone through menopause should get annual health checks, such as mammograms, bone density tests, and cholesterol checks, to keep an eye on and manage the increased risk of several conditions.

What can social and emotional support do for you?

Getting through menopause can be challenging, and help from family, friends, and support groups can be very helpful. Talking about their problems and how they deal with them can help you feel less alone.

Final Thoughts

In conclusion, menopause is a natural stage in a woman's life that causes significant changes in her hormones, which also affect many parts of her health. Understanding these changes is important to dealing with symptoms and maintaining a good quality of life during and after the shift. The problems that come with menopause can be improved by making changes to your lifestyle, seeking the right medical help, and leaning on support networks, all of which help women remain healthy and happy during this period.

2.5: CASE STUDIES: SUCCESSFUL HORMONAL BALANCE IN WOMEN OVER 40

For women over 40, maintaining hormonal balance is important for their health and well-being, as this is a time when significant hormonal shifts occur. This section highlights effective strategies and solutions for managing hormonal challenges in the adult population through various case studies. These real-life examples show women's problems and the best ways to deal with them to help them get through this time of life with ease and happiness.

Making Changes to Your Lifestyle to Deal With Menopause Symptoms

Background: At 52, Jane started having severe hot flashes, night sweats, and mood changes as she went through menopause. She looked for natural options for Hormone Replacement Therapy (HRT) because she was worried about the risks.

Her Approach: Jane focused on making changes to her habits, such as:

- **Diet**: Jane included phytoestrogens in foods like flaxseeds, soy products, and beans in her meals.
- **Doing regular exercise:** She committed to regular cardio and strength-training routines.
- **Stress Management:** Yoga and mindfulness meditation became her tools for managing stress.

Result: After six months, Jane noticed a significant reduction in her hot flashes and felt her mood was more stable. Her dedication to exercise also helped her sleep better and improved her overall energy levels.

Hormone Replacement Therapy for Signs of Severe Menopause

Background: Sarah, who is 48 years old, had terrible menopause symptoms like hot flashes and vaginal dryness that made her life and relationships difficult.

Her Approach: Sarah started a personalized HRT program after talking to her doctor. She will be closely watched to stay on track and deal with side effects.

Following the treatment, Sarah's problems got a lot better in just a few months. It also helped her deal with other problems that come with menopause, like losing bone structure.

How to Stop Weight Gain After Menopause

Background: At 55, Lisa found losing weight and maintaining it increasingly difficult post-menopause, which made her more likely to get diabetes and heart disease.

Her Approach

- **Changing her food:** Lisa switched to a Mediterranean diet, focusing on fruits, vegetables, whole grains, and healthy fats.
- **Physical Activity**: Walking every day and doing strength training.
- **Medical Consultation**: Regular check-ups for blood sugar and cholesterol levels were part of her plan.

Lisa not only lost weight, but she also said she had more energy and better control over her blood sugar levels, which made her less likely to get diabetes.

Dealing with the Mental and Emotional Effects of Hormonal Changes

Background: At 47, Anne faced mood swings and memory lapses that began to affect her daily life, both personally and professionally.

Her Approach: Anne's strategy included the following:

- **Emotional Support**: Anne sought therapy for her mood fluctuations and learned cognitive-behavioural skills to handle stress.
- **Cognitive Exercises**: She started engaging herself in activities like puzzles and memory games.
- **Nutritional Supplements**: She included B vitamins and omega-3 fatty acids in her routine to support brain health.

Over time, Anne's emotional state stabilized, and her cognitive functions, including memory, saw noticeable improvements, which improved her work and other personal relationships.

Natural Drugs to Keep Hormones in Balance

Background: At 43, Maria had to deal with irregular periods and the discomforts of premenstrual syndrome (PMS).

Her Approach:

- **Natural Supplements:** Maria chose natural supplements, such as **Vitex (Chasteberry)**, to control her periods.
- **Nutritional Support:** She further supplemented her diet with magnesium and Vitamin B6 to ease the symptoms of PMS.

Result: After a few months, Maria's periods became more regular, and her PMS symptoms, such as bloating and moodiness, got a lot better.

These case studies show that women over 40 can find more than one way to manage their hormonal changes effectively. Individualized methods that consider each person's health past and tastes are key to success, whether through lifestyle changes, medical treatments, or a combination of both. Getting help from doctors and focusing on your overall health is very important during this time of life, particularly when your hormones are changing.

GUT HEALTH MATTERS

"THE GREATEST WEALTH IS HEALTH." - VIRGIL

3.1: UNVEILING THE CRITICAL ROLE OF GUT HEALTH IN OVERALL WELLNESS

Even though it is essential for overall health, gut health is often overlooked. The gastrointestinal tract, more commonly known as the gut, is important for more than just digestion. It plays an important role in our mental health, immune system, and prevention of chronic diseases. This chapter goes into detail about why it's important to take care of our gut health and its role in influencing our overall health.

There is a second brain in the stomach.

Because the enteric nervous system comprises millions of nerves communicating directly with the brain, the gut is sometimes called the "second brain." This connection, known as the "gut-brain axis," suggests that the state of the gut can greatly affect mental health, influencing feelings of stress, depression, and anxiety.

Our Gut Microbiota and How It Influences Us

When it comes to health in general, the gut microbiome, which is composed of billions of bacteria, fungi, viruses, and other types of germs, is essential. These microbes play a key role in digesting food, extracting nutrients, and producing vitamins, such as B and K. Thus, maintaining a balanced gut microbiome is vital for proper bodily function and preventing dysbiosis—a condition where harmful bacteria outnumber the beneficial ones, leading to various health issues.

Maintaining a healthy immune system and gut is essential.

It's also essential to keep our immune system and gut in good health. Given that about 70% of the immune system resides in the gut, maintaining its health is essential for the body's defensive response. A healthy stomach allows the body to differentiate between potentially harmful and harmless intruders. As a result, inflammatory responses are stopped, and the likelihood of contracting infections and inflammation is reduced.

Their Role in the Prevention of Chronic Illnesses

Poor gut health is linked to several chronic conditions, including obesity, type 2 diabetes, cardiovascular disease, and certain cancers. For instance, an imbalance in the gut microbiome can lead to increased intestinal permeability or a "leaky gut." This condition allows toxins and pathogens to seep into the bloodstream, leading to inflammation and potentially worsening health issues.

Absorption of Nutrients and the Health of the Digestive Tract

The capacity of the digestive tract to absorb nutrients impacts overall health. A healthy gut lining makes it simpler for the body to absorb necessary nutrients, minerals, and vitamins. On the other hand, an unhealthy gut can lead to nutritional deficiencies, making it hard to maintain proper energy levels, bone health, and immune function.

Influences on One's Mental Health

Based on the gut-brain link, it is clear that a healthy gut may have a significant impact on mental health. Dopamine and serotonin are two neurotransmitters that are responsible for controlling mood and are produced by bacteria in the digestive tract. An imbalance in these bacteria can disrupt the production of these neurotransmitters, potentially leading to mental health issues.

Maintaining Your Weight and Maintaining the Health of Your Gut

Your digestion and weight are significantly impacted by the bacteria in your gut. There are specific kinds of germs that are more likely to be present in individuals who are overweight or obese, highlighting a correlation between gut health and weight management. These strains influence how food is broken down and how fat is stored in the body.

Here are some tips for maintaining a healthy gut:

- Consuming a wide variety of meals, particularly those rich in fiber, fermented foods, and prebiotics, is beneficial for maintaining healthy gut flora.

- Consuming foods or taking supplements rich in probiotics may help maintain a healthy balance of bacteria in the gut.
- Drinking plenty of water is important for maintaining the health of the mucous lining of the digestive tract.

Managing stress is extremely important because chronic stress negatively impacts gut health. Taking steps to reduce stress levels can be incredibly beneficial.

You **should not take antibiotics** when they are not required. Antibiotics should only be taken when necessary to avoid disrupting the balance of bacteria in your gut.

The Future of Gut Health Research

As more research is conducted on the bacteria in the gut and the gut-brain axis, we are gaining a better understanding of how maintaining a healthy gut may aid in preventing and treating disorders. Personalized diets and probiotic therapies are now being investigated in this research.

Final Thoughts

It may be concluded that gut health is an essential component of overall health since it impacts the immune system, the prevention of chronic illnesses, mental health, and the absorption of nutrients. It is essential to have a solid understanding of how to maintain a healthy stomach via diet, lifestyle choices, and medical treatments to ensure long-term health and well-being. The more research in this field, the greater the likelihood that novel therapies and techniques to prevent becoming sick will be developed. Thus, the importance of the gut in maintaining overall health cannot be overstated.

3.2: COMMON GUT-RELATED ISSUES AND THEIR IMPACT POST-40

By the time many of us hit forty, we might start to notice various digestive issues. These problems are not just about the occasional upset stomach; they can have broad implications for our health. Understanding these common digestive difficulties and recognizing their symptoms is key to keeping healthy as we age.

Rate of Metabolism That is Slower and Digesting That is Less Efficient

The problem is that the metabolism often slows down around the age of forty, and the digestive system might not work as well as it used to. This change can make it harder to digest certain foods, more difficult to absorb nutrients, and easier to gain weight.

As a result, a slower metabolism and digestive problems might cause you to gain weight, which in turn increases your risk of obesity and the health concerns that come along with it, such as type 2 diabetes and heart disease.

In Other Words, Gastroesophageal Reflux Disease (GERD)

Acid reflux disease (GERD), which includes heartburn and acid reflux, is increasingly prevalent in individuals as they get older. This condition happens when stomach acid flows back into the esophagus, the tube that links your mouth to the stomach.

Over time, gastroesophageal reflux disease (GERD) may cause discomfort and irritation in the throat. When it is severe enough, it may cause damage to the lining of the esophagus, which in turn increases the likelihood of developing esophageal cancer.

Intestinal dyspepsia is a frequent condition that affects the large intestine. Some of the symptoms it produces are cramps, stomach discomfort, bloating, gas, diarrhea, or difficulty reaching the restroom. It can become more prevalent as people age.

Although dyspepsia doesn't cause changes to bowel tissue or increase the risk of colon cancer, it can significantly make your life extremely difficult and lead you to feel uncomfortable, stressed out, and withdrawn from other people.

A Condition of Constipation

As people pass the age of 40, they're more likely to experience constipation, often because they do not exercise, eat poorly, and have changes in their gut motility (bowel movements).

Persistent constipation can lead to unpleasant conditions like hemorrhoids, anal fissures, and, in severe cases, fecal impaction. Besides its physical effects, constipation can also contribute to anxiety and stress, affecting your mental health.

A Condition That Affects the Diverticular Canal

People who suffer from this condition have diverticula, which are like tiny holes in their digestive tract. These tiny holes develop due to the weakening of the gut wall, a change that often comes with age.

Most of the time, diverticula don't cause any trouble. But if they become infected or inflamed, they can lead to diverticulitis, and you will notice symptoms such as severe abdominal pain, fever, and digestive disturbances.

Alterations in the Microbiota That Populate the Gut

As people get older, the number of different bacteria that live in their guts may decrease, which can lead to an imbalance known as dysbiosis. Changes in nutrition, decreased physical activity, or certain uses of medication might make this condition worse.

Indicators: Dysbiosis can have several negative effects on health, including a diminished immune system, increased inflammation, an increased risk of developing gastrointestinal disorders, and even mental health issues.

The risk of developing stomach ulcers and Gastritis is significantly increased.

With age, the risk of developing gastric ulcers and gastritis also goes up. Additionally, the use of non-steroidal anti-inflammatory drugs (NSAIDs) for an extended period or the presence of H. pylori bacteria in the stomach may make the condition even more severe.

Gastritic ulcers can cause severe abdominal pain and bleeding. You must get medical attention as soon as possible since, in severe instances, they can lead to perforations in the stomach wall.

The Likelihood of Developing Colorectal Cancer

As the risk of colorectal cancer increases significantly after the age of 40, it is essential to undergo annual screenings every year.

Effect: The early detection of colon cancer is critical for successfully treating the disease. Failure to undergo screening may result in a late diagnosis, making the cancer harder to treat and potentially life-threatening.

Final Thoughts

The takeaway is clear: people over 40 often face digestive issues that can significantly affect their overall health and quality of life. Individuals need to be aware of these potential problems and take proactive steps to address them. Some steps they can take include adjusting their diet, engaging in regular physical activity, reducing their stress levels, and going to the doctor for regular check-ups. The first step in reducing the effects of these common gut disorders and maintaining a healthy and active lifestyle as you age is to educate yourself.

3.3: GUT HEALTH, INFLAMMATION, AND THE IMMUNE SYSTEM

Keeping your immune system strong, keeping your gut healthy, and controlling inflammation are important for your overall health. This synergy is especially important for people over 40, since getting older can affect these processes differently. Understanding this relationship is essential for a long, healthy life with a strong immune system.

Gut Health and Why It's Important

The gut, which is also called the gastrointestinal (GI) tract, stretches from the mouth to the anus and plays a key role in processing food, absorbing nutrients, and shielding the body from harmful substances. Over time, it has evolved to perform another important role: it now houses a vast and diverse group of gut microbiota.

Gut Microbiota: There are trillions of germs living in the gut, such as bacteria, viruses, fungi, and more. This microbiome is important for many bodily functions, such as digestion, metabolism, and keeping the defense system in check.

Inflammation and the Two Sides of It

Redness, swelling, heat, and pain are all signs of inflammation, which is a fundamental aspect of the body's defense system. This is how the body protects itself from getting sick, hurt, and other threats. However, inflammation can also be a double-edged sword: it can both help and hurt cells.

- **Acute Inflammation**: This is the body's immediate response to being hurt or infected. Its goal is to eliminate the danger, fix damaged cells, and get things back to normal. Acute inflammation is a managed process that lasts for a short time.
- **Chronic Inflammation**: When inflammation persists over a long period, it becomes chronic. Chronic inflammation can be caused by a bad diet, not moving around much, stress, and pre-existing health conditions. It is linked to a lot of different diseases, like heart disease, diabetes, and inflammatory illnesses.

This is the gut-immune system axis.

There are several things in the gut that affect how the immune system works, and they all work together to do this:

GALT stands for "gut-associated lymphoid tissue." The GI tract is home to GALT, it's an important part of the defense system. It has tonsils, lymph nodes, and Peyer's patches in it. GALT's job is to keep an eye on possible threats in the gut, like bacteria or dangerous chemicals, and respond to these potential threats.

- **Interaction between bacteria and the immune system**: The microbiota in the gut communicates with the immune system. A healthy, guilty gut keeps your immune system in balance. On the other hand, dysbiosis (an imbalance of microbes) can cause inflammation and immune system problems.

The covering of the gut keeps dangerous chemicals from getting into the bloodstream. This is called the mucosal barrier. Damage to the gut lining can lead to increased inflammation and immune responses.

Changes and Effects Caused by Aging

As we age, the relationship between gut health, inflammation, and the immune system goes through significant changes.

- **Changes in Gut bacteria:** Older people's gut bacteria may differ. This can lead to a less varied microbiome, linked to more inflammation and a weaker immune system.
- **Aging of the Immune System:** The immune system gets older, which is called immunosenescence, and can make the immune system less effective. This can reduce your body's ability to fight off infections and increase your risk of developing chronic inflammation problems.
- **Inflammation and Aging**: A condition called inflammaging describes how chronic inflammation worsens with age. Low-level, long-lasting inflammation is a major cause of illnesses and weakness that come with getting older.

What It Means for Women Over 40

Because of the changes in hormones during perimenopause and menopause, women over 40 should know how gut health, inflammation, and the immune system affect each other. Hormonal changes during this time can influence gut bacteria and immune function, which could make problems related to inflammation even worse.

- **Affects Hormones:** Estrogen, a very important hormone for women, has been shown to change gut bacteria and immune reactions. Lower estrogen levels during menopause can worsen gut dysbiosis and change how the immune system functions.
- **Immune Resilience**: For women over 40, maintaining their gut health and controlling inflammation is key to strengthening their immune systems. Some possible solutions are a healthy diet, regular exercise, learning how to deal with stress, and taking probiotics.

Final Thoughts

In conclusion, the link between gut health, inflammation, and the immune system plays an important role in determining overall health, especially for people over 40 and women experiencing hormonal changes. A healthy diet, exercise, lowering stress, and encouraging a diverse gut flora are all part of an overall approach that can help keep your immune system strong and lessen the adverse effects of chronic inflammation. Understanding this complex relationship gives people the power to make choices that will improve their health and well-being as they age.

Here is a table to summarize the information about the relationship between gut health, inflammation, and the immune system:

Aspect	Description
Gut Health Significance	The gut is a complex system that functions in digestion and nutrient absorption. It houses trillions of microorganisms, known as the gut microbiota, which are essential for various processes.
Inflammation Nature	Inflammation can be both protective (acute inflammation) and detrimental (chronic inflammation). Chronic inflammation is associated with various diseases.
Gut-Immune System Axis	The gut modulates the immune system through components like GALT, microbiota-immune interaction, and the mucosal barrier.
Age-Related Changes	Aging can influence gut microbiota, and immune system function and lead to chronic inflammation (inflammaging).
Impact on Women Over 40	Hormonal changes during menopause can affect gut health and immune function and exacerbate inflammation-related issues.
Hormonal Influence	Reduced estrogen levels during menopause can contribute to gut dysbiosis and altered immune function.

Immune Resilience Strategies	Maintaining a healthy gut and managing inflammation becomes essential for supporting immune resilience in women over 40.
Holistic Approach	A holistic approach includes a balanced diet, regular exercise, stress management, and probiotics to promote immune resilience.
Conclusion	Understanding the gut-inflammation-immune system connection empowers individuals to make informed choices for better health.

This table provides a concise summary of the key points regarding the relationship between gut health, inflammation, and the immune system, with a specific focus on its impact on women over 40.

3.4: PROBIOTICS, PREBIOTICS, AND DIET: KEYS TO A HEALTHY GUT

Maintaining a healthy gut is essential for overall health, particularly for women over 40. A healthy and well-balanced gut is strongly linked to the ability to digest food effectively, absorb nutrients, and maintain a robust defense system. The upcoming section will explore how probiotics, prebiotics, and food choices can help you maintain a healthy gut.

In addition to The Beneficial Bacteria

Live microorganisms, mostly bacteria and certain yeasts, are known as probiotics. Adding sufficient amounts of probiotics to your diet might be beneficial to your health. These good bacteria are found in fermented foods and beverages such as yogurt, kefir, sauerkraut, kimchi, and probiotics can also be taken as supplements.

For the health of the gut, probiotics are particularly helpful in several ways, including the following:

- **Maintaining a Balanced Gut Microbiota:** Probiotics are immensely helpful in maintaining a diverse and balanced microbiota in the gut. They increase the number of beneficial bacteria, which can outcompete harmful ones, thereby reducing the chances of dysbiosis—a microbial imbalance.
- **Aids Digestion:** Certain bacteria help break down complex meals, facilitating the absorption of essential nutrients, including vitamins and minerals.
- **Supports the Immune System:** The gut-associated lymphoid tissue (GALT), a significant immune system component, is the third organ that probiotics interact with. They are essential since the immune system manages defensive responses that protect you.
- **Reducing inflammation:** Certain probiotics produce molecules that have anti-inflammatory properties, which may help reduce chronic inflammation, particularly in women over 40.
- **Improves Mental Health:** Recent research highlights a link between gut health and mental well-being. Taking probiotics may make you happier and reduce feelings of anxiety and depression.

Probiotics need prebiotics as their source of nutrition.

Probiotics are edible grains that cannot be broken down, yet they nourish probiotics and other beneficial bacteria in the digestive tract. They are found in a variety of plant-based foods, including:

- **Fruits:** Bananas, apples, and berries contain prebiotic fibers. Inulin and oligofructose are two examples of it.
- **Vegetables:** Foods rich in veggies, such as artichokes, garlic, onions, leeks, and asparagus, are excellent prebiotic sources.
- **Whole Grains:** Beta-glucans are a kind of prebiotic fiber that may be found in whole grains, such as oats and barley.
- **Legumes:** Certain legumes, such as chickpeas, lentils, and beans, are excellent providers of prebiotics.

Prebiotics feed the probiotics in the gut, helping them develop and spread throughout the gut. The interaction between prebiotics and probiotics is of the utmost significance for maintaining a healthy balance of bacteria in the gut.

What to Consume to Maintain Gut Health

Women over 40 should focus on eating a wide variety of meals to maintain a healthy digestive tract. **Here are some recommendations for maintaining gut health:**

- **High-Fiber Foods:** Make sure to eat plenty of fiber-rich foods, including whole grains, fruits, vegetables, and beans. Fiber is great for the bacteria in your gut and helps keep your bowel movements regular.
- **Fermented Foods:** Kombucha, kefir, kimchi, and yogurt are all examples of fermented foods that you should consume. In their natural state, these foods contain a significant amount of probiotics.
- **Lean Proteins:** When looking for a meat substitute, pick lean protein sources such as fish, poultry, and plant-based proteins. This may reduce the consumption of fatty lipids, which are detrimental to the health of your digestive tract.
- **Healthy Fats:** Consuming foods rich in healthy fats, such as avocados, nuts, seeds, and olive oil. These fats not only support overall health but also help your body absorb fat-soluble vitamins.
- **Limit Processed and Sugary Foods:** Foods that are highly processed and heavy in sugar should be consumed in moderation since they have the potential to disrupt the natural balance of bacteria in the gut and lead to inflammation.
- **Stay Hydrated:** Drink enough water to keep your body hydrated and aid in meal digestion. This will also help maintain the health of the mucous layer in your stomach.
- **Avoid Alcohol and Caffeine Intake:** Too much caffeine can irritate your intestinal walls, so moderation is key.
- **Manage Your Stress:** Chronic stress may be detrimental to your stomach's health. Finding ways to alleviate stress through daily practices like yoga,

meditation, or mindfulness can offer significant
relief.

In summary, the foods women over 40 choose to eat, along
with incorporating probiotics and prebiotics, are all essential
for maintaining the health of their digestive tracts. Adding
these practices to your daily routine can benefit your gut,
boost your immune system, lessen inflammation, and
improve your overall health. Remember, taking care of your
gut is essential to achieving the highest possible state of
health.

3.5: STEP-BY-STEP GUIDE TO REVITALIZING GUT HEALTH

Gut health restoration is a life-changing process that significantly impacts overall health, especially for women over 40.
This step-by-step guide provides methods and tips for taking
care of your gut and returning it to its best state. Doing these
things can improve your stomach, boost your immune
system, lower inflammation, and make you feel more
energetic.

Look at what you eat and how you live now.

To improve your gut health, you should first look at
what you eat and how you live. Look closely at how you
eat, how active you are, how stressed you are, and how
you sleep. Find things that might be causing gut problems, like eating too many processed foods, being
stressed out, or not getting enough sleep. Figuring out
where you started is very important for making changes
that work.

Eat foods that are good for your gut.

Adding foods that help keep gut bacteria healthy is important to restoring gut health. Pay attention to these things:

- **Fiber:** Eat more whole grains, fruits, veggies, beans,
  and other foods high in fiber. Fiber is prebiotic,
  which means it feeds good bacteria in the gut.
- **Probiotics**: Eat fermented foods like kimchi, yogurt,
  kefir, and cabbage. Probiotics are good for gut health
  and can be found naturally in these foods.
- **Prebiotics**: Eat foods high in prebiotics, such as
  garlic, onions, leeks, and asparagus, to feed and help
  the growth of probiotics.
- **Lean Proteins**: To reduce excess fat, choose lean
  protein sources like chicken, fish, and plant-based
  proteins.
- **Healthy Fats:** To get the most nutrients, eat healthy
  fats like bananas, nuts, seeds, and olive oil.

Drink plenty of water and avoid irritants.

Getting enough water is important for good health. It helps
keep the gut's mucous layer in good shape and makes digestion easier. But watch out for allergens like too much coffee
and booze, which can damage the gut lining. Moderation is
key when having these drinks.

Deal with stress.

Long-term stress can harm gut health. To lower your stress
levels, use methods for dealing with stress, like yoga, meditation, deep breathing movements, or awareness. Rest and self-
care are also important for gut regeneration.

Make good sleep a priority.

A good night's sleep is important for both general and gut health. Aim for 7 to 9 hours of quality sleep each night. To get better sleep, set a regular sleep plan and make a relaxing habit before bed.

Make changes to your diet slowly.

If you want to improve your gut health by changing your diet, do it slowly. Sudden changes can lead to discomfort, such as stomach pain. Over time, make changes that will last. For example, slowly eat more fiber and fermented foods.

Keep an eye on and pay attention to your body.

Watch how your body reacts to changes in your diet and lifestyle. Keep a diary to write down any changes for the better or worse. If you have stomach problems or bad reactions to certain foods, talk to a doctor or nurse for advice.

Consider taking probiotic supplements.

Probiotic pills may help sometimes, especially if you have certain gut health problems. Talk to your doctor or nurse to determine what probiotics you should take and how much.

Get help from a professional.

If you have ongoing gut health problems or think there may be a more serious issue, you should see a doctor. A doctor or trained dietitian can look at your case, tell you what tests you might need, and give you personalized help.

Keep being consistent and patient.

Restoring gut health is a journey that takes time and determination. It may take some time for your gut health to improve, so staying committed to your process is important. Celebrate the little wins along the way, like better digestion, more energy, and better health in general.

Restoring gut health is an all-around approach to health that can have a huge effect on the lives of women over 40. By following this step-by-step guide, you can take charge of your gut health and achieve the best possible state of health. Remember that everyone's journey is different, so pay close attention to your body and get help from a professional when needed. If this journey of change sparks excitement in you, you're on track to discovering a better, more energetic you.

THE ENERGY EQUATION

"LET FOOD BE THY MEDICINE AND MEDICINE BE THY FOOD." - HIPPOCRATES

4.1: DECODING THE DECLINE IN ENERGY LEVELS POST-40

E nergy is the source of power for both our physical and mental actions, and that's why energy is an essential component of our day-to-day lives. However, many women notice a drop in their energy levels once they hit their forties and beyond. This decline can significantly affect overall health and quality of life. Suppose we want to find a solution to this issue successfully. In that case, it's important to understand the causes of decreased energy in people over 40 and explore ways to boost energy levels after this age.

Having an Understanding of the Energy Decrease

After age forty, women often experience a decline in their energy levels, which may be attributed to several interconnected variables. The following are some of these factors:

- **Changes in Hormones:** One of the primary reasons women experience a decrease in their energy levels beyond 40 is changes in their hormones, particularly the decrease in estrogen and progesterone during perimenopause and menopause. Hormones govern how your body utilizes energy, and when they are out of balance, you may experience feelings of fatigue.
- **Alterations in metabolism:** As individuals age, their metabolism slows. Because of this, the body burns fewer calories when it is not actively engaged in any activity. This might cause you to feel weary and cause you to gain weight. Alterations in the strength of muscles may also affect metabolism.
- **Increased Likelihood of Sleep Disruptions:** Women are more prone to sleep disruptions as they age, especially older women. Changes in hormone levels, hot flashes, and night sweats may make it difficult to fall asleep, resulting in fatigue and sluggishness throughout the day.
- **Lifestyle and Stress:** Women over 40 may experience higher stress levels due to their increased responsibilities at work and with their children. Stress that persists for an extended period of time may deplete their energy and leave them feeling exhausted.
- **Nutritional Deficiencies:** Iron, B vitamins, and calcium are all examples of nutritional deficiencies that inadequate nutrition, poor dietary choices, or difficulties with intake may cause. These shortcomings may cause fatigue and a decrease in energy.

- **Failure to engage in physical activity:** If you don't move about too much, your muscles may weaken, and your energy may decrease, which will cause you to feel even more exhausted.

Boosting Your Energy Levels After the Age of 40

Even though experiencing a decline in energy levels is a natural consequence of aging, there are a few things that you can do to maintain your health and combat fatigue:

- **The Management of Hormones:** Discuss the possibility of hormone replacement therapy (HRT) or natural methods of addressing hormonal disorders with your primary care physician. Taking care of your hormones may assist with a variety of symptoms, including feeling sleepy.
- **Regular Exercise:** Exercising regularly increases your energy levels, develops your muscles, and speeds up your metabolism. Aerobics and strength training are examples of exercises that fall into this category.
- **Balanced Diet:** Consume a meal rich in various foods, including lean meats, fruits, vegetables, whole grains, and healthy fats. Take vitamins if you feel the need to compensate for any nutritional deficiencies.
- **Quality Sleep:** Develop healthy sleeping habits and create an environment conducive to sleep. If necessary, talk to a healthcare physician about your sleep difficulties.
- **Stress Management:** Find stress-relieving activities that work for you, such as yoga, meditation,

mindfulness, or deep breathing exercises.

- **Hydration:** Drink a large amount of water during the day; if you are dehydrated, you may experience fatigue. Only a small amount of coffee should be consumed, particularly in the afternoon and evening.
- **Regular Health Checkups:** Schedule regular appointments with your healthcare provider to screen for any underlying conditions that may be causing your fatigue. The need to address these issues as soon as possible cannot be overstated.
- **Mind-Body Practices:** Exercises focusing on the mind and body, such as tai chi or qigong, may help you enhance your energy flow and overall health.
- **Strong Support Network:** Having a solid network of friends and family members is important since positive relationships can significantly benefit your mental and emotional well-being.
- **Time Management:** Effectively manage your time by planning your day, prioritizing tasks by importance, and scheduling time to rest and take care of yourself.

The decrease in energy experienced by women over 40 can be influenced by various factors. This does not mean that women must accept that they will always be exhausted, even though feeling tired is a natural aspect of growing older. By identifying the factors contributing to their energy levels and taking steps to address them, women may take control of their energy levels and live a more energetic and fulfilling life well into their forties and beyond.

4.2: HOW INFLAMMATION AND HORMONES AFFECT ENERGY

Energy is an important resource that drives everything, from moving around to thinking. It gives us the energy to do what we need every day, enjoy what we love, and stay healthy. On the other hand, the complicated relationship between inflammation and hormones can have a big effect on energy levels, especially in women over 40. You need to know how these affect your energy to be as healthy and energetic as possible.

The body's alarm system is inflamed.

Inflammation is a normal and important immune system reaction that keeps the body safe from harm, such as pain, infection, or other dangerous things. Pro-inflammatory cytokines are messaging molecules that initiate the immune reaction when the body senses a threat. This short-term inflammation is very important for healing and protecting against germs.

But problems start when inflammation lasts for a long time. It can happen when the defense system stays active, even when there is no threat. Several health problems, such as autoimmune diseases, heart disease, and cancer, are linked to chronic inflammation. In addition, it has a big effect on how much energy you have.

What happens to energy when you have chronic inflammation?

Chronic inflammation stresses the body, taking resources away from important processes, which further makes people tired and low on energy. Here's how it impacts energy levels:

- **Diversion of Energy**: When the body has continuous inflammation, it uses energy and resources to keep the inflammatory reaction going. This takes energy away from other important body processes, resulting in tiredness and lethargy.
- **Trouble sleeping:** People with chronic inflammation often have trouble sleeping. Some diseases, like arthritis and inflammatory bowel disease, can cause pain and discomfort, making it hard to sleep. Inflammation can also change the parts of the brain that control sleep, making it impossible to sleep or making your sleep less restful.
- **Muscle Fatigue**: Molecules that cause inflammation can directly affect muscle tissue, making muscles tired and weak. This can make you feel physically tired and lower your energy.
- **Mental Fatigue**: Long-term inflammation can make it hard to think clearly, causing what is commonly called "brain fog." People may have trouble focusing, remembering things, and thinking clearly, making them feel less energetic.

Hormones are like pacemakers for energy.

Hormones are chemical messages important for controlling how our bodies use energy. Hormonal changes happen all the time in women, but they are especially noticeable during puberty, pregnancy, and menopause. Estrogen and progesterone are the two primary hormones that affect how much energy you have.

- **Estrogen:** It is known that estrogen affects energy directly. Estrogen amounts go up and down with the monthly cycle, which affects energy levels. During the luteal phase (when estrogen levels drop), many women say they feel more tired, while during the follicular phase (when estrogen levels rise), they feel more energized and mentally sharp.
- **Progesterone:** Another female sex hormone, progesterone, can also change how much energy you have. This hormone can cause ease and sleepiness because it calms the nervous system.

How Hormones and Inflammation Work Together

Hormones and inflammation are linked in a complicated way. Long-term inflammation can throw off hormonal balance, which can further complicate energy problems. For example:

- **Hormonal Imbalances:** Long-term inflammation can mess up how hormones are made and controlled. It can cause problems like polycystic ovary syndrome (PCOS) or thyroid issues, which can often make you feel tired.

- **Hormonal Fluctuations:** Inflammation can make the signs of hormonal changes, such as those that happen during perimenopause and menopause, worse. Mood changes, hot flashes, and night sweats can make sleeping hard and contribute to tiredness.
- **Insulin Resistance:** Insulin resistance is when the body's cells don't respond properly to insulin. It is linked to chronic inflammation. This can cause changes in blood sugar levels, resulting in tiredness and energy drops.

How to Keep Hormones and Inflammation in Check

To properly control energy levels, dealing with both inflammation and chemical issues is important. Here are some approaches:

- **Anti-inflammatory Diet:** Eating many fruits, veggies, whole grains, and healthy fats can help lower chronic inflammation.
- **Regular Exercise:** Regular exercise can help reduce inflammation and keep hormones balanced.
- **Dealing with stress:** Long-term stress can worsen inflammation and chemical issues. Techniques for lowering stress, like yoga and meditation, can be helpful.
- **Hormone Management:** Talking to your doctor about hormone replacement treatment (HRT) or exploring natural solutions for hormonal imbalances can be effective.
- **Quality Sleep**: Prioritizing good sleep hygiene and making your bedroom a relaxing place for

comfortable sleep.
- **Nutritional Supplements:** For nutritional support, consider taking anti-inflammatory products like ginger, omega-3 fatty acids, and adaptogenic plants.

In summary, the complex link between inflammation and hormones can significantly impact the energy levels of women over 40. Long-term inflammation wastes energy and interferes with important bodily processes. Changing hormones can also cause energy-related complaints. Women can control their energy levels and live a vibrant, active life as they age by learning how inflammation and hormones work together and taking steps to keep them in balance.

4.3: NUTRITIONAL STRATEGIES TO BOOST ENERGY

Women over 40 need to pay special attention to their diet to stay healthy and live a fulfilling life. During this time in life, the body goes through many changes, such as changes in hormones and metabolism. Because of these changes, it is important to follow certain eating habits to maintain your energy levels and overall health. Here are some key health factors and tips to help women over 40 boost and sustain their energy:

Keeping the Macronutrients in Check

- **Complex Carbohydrates:** Whole grains, beans, and veggies are all great sources of complex carbohydrates, which give you energy that lasts for a long time. They slowly release glucose into the bloodstream, which keeps energy levels steady throughout the day and stops energy crashes. Fiber-rich foods, like oats and brown rice, are especially good for you.

- **Lean Proteins**: Protein is important for keeping muscle mass, which is important for burning calories. Adding lean protein sources like chicken, fish, tofu, and beans can help keep your energy levels steady. Protein-rich snacks can also help you feel fuller without overeating.
- **Healthy Fats**: Omega-3 fatty acids found in fatty fish, flaxseeds, and walnuts are essential for brain health and reducing inflammation. Adding these healthy fats to your diet can help your brain work better and provide longer-lasting energy.

Taking Care of Blood Sugar

- **Eat regular meals and snacks**. Skipping meals can lead to fluctuations in blood sugar levels and result in energy drops. You need to eat meals and snacks at regular, consistent times to keep your blood sugar levels steady. Try to snack on healthy foods like whole-grain bread with almond butter or yogurt with berries.
- **Limiting added sugars:** Eating too much sugar can cause blood sugar to rise and fall quickly. Reducing sugary drinks, candies, and processed foods can help you keep your energy level steady all day.
- **Be aware of the glycemic index (GI).** The glycemic index (GI) measures how quickly carbohydrates in foods raise blood sugar levels. Choosing foods with a

lower GI can provide you with energy that lasts longer as they are digested more slowly. Eat low-GI foods, like sweet potatoes, rice, and beans.

Support for Micronutrients

- **Vitamins and Minerals**: Getting enough vitamins and minerals is important for making energy. The B-complex vitamins—B1, B2, B3, B5, B6, B7, B9, and B12—are very important for turning food into energy. Iron and magnesium are two minerals that are also involved in energy production.
- **Antioxidants**: Foods high in antioxidants, such as nuts, berries, and spinach, help protect cells from toxic stress. Lowering reactive stress can make you healthier and give you more energy.

Drinking Water

- **Right Hydration**: Being dehydrated can make you feel tired and less alert. Staying refreshed by drinking water, herbal teas, and water-rich foods, like watermelon, can help you keep your energy up.

Planned Meal Times

- **Balanced Breakfast:** Eating a well-balanced breakfast with healthy fats, complex carbs, and proteins can boost your metabolism and give you energy all day.
- **Lighter Dinners:** You can sleep better if you eat a light dinner and avoid eating heavy meals close to

bedtime. Getting more sleep can help you have more energy during the day.

Supplements

- **Think About Supplements**: Dietary supplements may be helpful in some situations. Women over 40 should talk to a healthcare provider about their unique needs. Vitamin D, calcium, and gut bacteria are common nutrients for gut health.

Personalized Method

- **Personalized Nutrition:** It's important to understand that everyone has different dietary needs. Genetics, amount of exercise, and underlying health problems are some of the things that affect which diet is most suitable for them. Talking to a trained dietitian can give you specific advice.

Final Thoughts

Nutrition plays a key role in maintaining energy levels and overall health, particularly for women over 40. Women can maintain their energy levels by adding a diet rich in complex carbohydrates, lean proteins, and healthy fats, carefully managing blood sugar, ensuring there are enough micronutrients, staying well-hydrated, and being mindful of meal timings. To get the most out of their energy and live a fulfilling, busy life as they age, it's extremely important to treat eating as a personal matter and seek help when needed.

Here's a table summarizing the key nutritional strategies to boost energy for women over 40:

Nutritional Strategy	Description
Complex Carbohydrates	Include whole grains, legumes, and vegetables for sustained energy.
Lean Proteins	Incorporate sources like poultry, fish, tofu, and legumes to maintain muscle mass and energy metabolism.
Healthy Fats	Omega-3 fatty acids from fatty fish, flaxseeds, and walnuts support brain health and sustained energy.
Regular Meals and Snacks	Avoid skipping meals and enjoy balanced snacks to keep blood sugar levels stable.
Limiting Added Sugars	Reduce consumption of sugary beverages, candies, and processed foods to prevent energy crashes.
Glycemic Index Awareness	Opt for low-GI foods like sweet potatoes, quinoa, and lentils to provide sustained energy.
Vitamins and Minerals	Ensure adequate intake of B-complex vitamins, iron, and magnesium for energy production.
Antioxidants	Consume antioxidant-rich foods like berries and nuts to reduce oxidative stress and improve energy levels.

Proper Hydration	Stay hydrated with water, herbal teas, and hydrating foods like watermelon to prevent fatigue.
Balanced Breakfast	Start the day with a balanced breakfast to kickstart your metabolism and provide sustained energy.
Lighter Dinners	Opt for lighter dinners and avoid heavy, rich meals close to bedtime for better sleep quality and energy during the day.
Consideration of Supplements	Discuss specific supplement needs with a healthcare provider, including vitamin D, calcium, and probiotics for gut health.
Personalized Nutrition	Recognize individual nutritional needs and seek guidance from a registered dietitian for a tailored approach.

These strategies can help women over 40 optimize their energy levels and overall well-being through proper nutrition.

4.4: ROLE OF SLEEP AND REST IN ENERGY MANAGEMENT

Sleeping and resting are crucial for managing energy, especially for women over 40. As we age, our bodies undergo many changes that affect how we sleep and how much energy we have. To live a healthy and active lifestyle at this point in your life, you need to know how important sleep and rest are for managing your energy.

1. What Does Sleep Do for Energy

How You Sleep Changes as You Age

One big change that women over 40 may notice is that their sleep habits may change. People this age often have trouble falling asleep or feeling better after a night of lighter, more scattered sleep. Hormonal changes are often to blame for these changes, especially in women who are nearing or have already gone through menopause.

Hormones and What They Do

Hormones like estrogen and progesterone are very important for controlling when you sleep and wake up. As women go through perimenopause and menopause, their hormone levels drop. This can mess up their circadian schedule, making it harder for them to get a good night's sleep. This sort of disruption can make you tired and less energetic throughout the day.

Why Deep Sleep is Important

Deep sleep, sometimes called slow-wave sleep, is an important stage for recharging your batteries and improving your health. This is an important time for the body to do important things like fix damaged tissues, build muscle, and make memories stronger. Deep sleep tends to get less deep as people get older, which makes it harder for the body to heal and recharge.

How Well You Sleep is Important

Not just how long your sleep is important; how well you sleep is also very important. Snoring, sleep apnea, or waking up often during the night can all be caused by bad sleep quality. All of these problems can throw off the sleep cycle. Regularly waking up or having bad sleep can make you feel groggy and give you less energy during the day.

2. How Sleep Can Help You Feel Better

Conservation of Energy

One way to think about sleep is as a time when the body saves and recovers energy. While in deep sleep, the body's metabolism rate slows down, which means it needs less energy. By conserving energy, the body can refuel itself, which makes you feel refreshed and ready to go in the morning.

Brain Function

Getting enough sleep is very important for brain functions like remembering, focus, and problem-solving. Cognitive ability decreases when you don't get enough sleep, and jobs that require focus and mental clarity become harder. This can make you feel mentally tired and give you less energy overall.

Good Mental Health

Good sleep is closely linked to emotional health. When you don't get enough sleep, mood problems like restlessness, worry, and sadness can occur. These mental problems can

THE ENERGY EQUATION | 93

drain your energy even more, making it hard to enjoy the things you do every day.

Ways to Get Better Rest and Sleep

Because sleep and rest are so important for keeping your energy up, women over 40 need to do the following to get better sleep:

- **Good sleep habits**

Good sleep hygiene includes maintaining a regular sleep routine, making your bedroom comfy, and avoiding exciting activities before bedtime.

- **Dealing with stress**

Stress can make it hard to sleep. Meditation, deep breathing routines, and yoga are good ways to reduce stress and help you rest and sleep better.

- **Getting regular exercise**

Regular exercise can help you sleep better and keep your sleep habits in check. But don't do a lot of intense exercise right before bed because it might keep you awake.

- **A well-balanced diet**

A well-balanced diet can help you sleep better. Eat light or hot meals before bed, and drink less booze and coffee, especially in the evening.

- **Talk to a medical professional.**

If you still can't sleep, you should see a doctor to rule out any underlying health problems or to talk about possible hormone treatment choices for menopause symptoms that make it harder to fall asleep.

To sum up, sleep and rest are important parts of managing energy for women over 40. Acknowledging that sleep patterns evolve with age and actively taking steps to improve the quality of your sleep can have a big effect on your overall energy, mental health, and emotional well-being. Priortizing good sleep habits first and getting professional help when needed can make a big difference in living a better and more energetic life at this point in your life.

4.5: REAL-LIFE TIPS FOR SUSTAINING HIGH ENERGY LEVELS

For many women over forty, maintaining their energy levels is a goal. While aging is the natural cause of some physical changes, there are practical solutions that can improve your everyday life and even help you increase your energy levels. These tips cover many areas of your everyday life, from what you eat and how much you exercise to dealing with stress and making choices about your lifestyle. Making these habits a part of your daily life will make you feel more alive and energetic.

Food to Give You Energy:

- **Varied Diet:** For long-lasting energy, you need to eat a varied diet. Ensure your meals include foods from all the food groups, such as veggies, fruits, whole grains, healthy fats, and lean meats. This gives your body the nutrients it needs to make energy.

- **Regular Meals:** Skipping meals can tire you, so don't do it. Eat smaller meals more often during the day to keep your blood sugar levels steady and avoid energy crashes.
- **Hydration**: Being dehydrated can make you tired and low on energy. Drink plenty of water throughout the day to stay properly hydrated. You can also choose herbal drinks or water with added flavors to cool you down.
- **Limit Sugar and Processed Foods**: Consuming a lot of sugar and processed foods can cause rapid fluctuations in your energy levels. Limit the consumption of sugary snacks and processed foods you eat. Instead, choose whole, raw foods.

Do Some Physical Activity:

- **Daily Exercise:** Physical exercise is one of the best ways to get more energy. Exercise increases blood flow, provides cells with more oxygen, and builds overall strength. Power training and aerobics should both be part of your practice.
- **"Morning Workouts":** Try working out in the morning. It can speed up your metabolism and give you energy that lasts all day.
- **Stay Active During the Day:** Find ways to move around besides your planned workouts. Instead of sitting for long amounts of time, go for short walks, use a standing desk, or do stretching activities.

Taking Care of Stress:

- **Tips for Reducing Worry**: Long-term worry can make you tired. Try to calm your mind and lower stress through yoga, awareness, meditation, deep breathing routines, or meditation.
- **Adequate Sleep**: Get enough good sleep to regain energy. Set up a relaxing routine before bed, and try to get between 7 and 9 hours of sleep each night.

Choices for a Lifestyle:

- **Limit Caffeine and Alcohol**: Drinking too much caffeine and alcohol can make it hard to sleep and give you energy swings. Limit how much of these drinks you can drink, especially in the hours before bed.
- **Social Connections**: Keep in touch with people and do things you love. Hobbies and relationships with positive people can make you feel better and boost your energy.
- **Set Realistic Goals**: Avoid overloading yourself with too many tasks. Schedule only a few chores and responsibilities. Make attainable goals and organize your tasks so you stay energized.

Link Between Mind and Body:

- **Mindfulness and Gratitude**: Being more aware and showing gratitude can improve your outlook on life. You're likely to feel more lively and full of life when you pay attention to the present and appreciate what you have right now.

- **Positive Self-Talk**: Keep an eye on your thoughts and replace the negative ones with positive affirmations. Staying positive can help you feel more energetic.

Regular Checkups With a Doctor:

- **Regular Checkups**: To monitor your health, make an appointment with your doctor for regular checkups. Take care of any underlying health problems or hormonal issues that might be draining your energy.

Pay Attention to Your Body:

- **Rest When Needed**: Know how important it is to rest and heal. Don't feel guilty about taking breaks if you're feeling tired.
- **Stay in touch with your body:** Tune in to what your body is saying. If you always feel tired or have other unusual symptoms, make sure to consult a doctor for a full evaluation.

To sum up, women over 40 can maintain high energy levels by paying attention to their diet, exercise, how they handle stress, lifestyle choices, and self-care. You can boost your energy, improve your general health, and live a more fulfilling and lively life by making these real-life tips a part of your daily routine and way of life. Remember that making small changes over time can significantly impact your health and energy.

Embracing the Years You've Been in Training For

"There will always be someone who can't see your worth. Don't let it be you."

— MEL ROBBINS

How did you feel about turning 40? For the majority of women in their 30s, the idea of that big birthday brings a feeling of dread and prompts a host of reflections. Perhaps you thought about all the things you'd hoped to have achieved by this stage in life; maybe you compared yourself to your parents when they were turning 40; perhaps you started worrying about your health or the shape your body was in.

It's true that things start to change as we enter our 40s and 50s, but that dread that we feel when we're younger is born out of nothing more than worry and comparison. Your best years aren't behind you… In fact, they're still to come. You've been in training for them your whole life, so now isn't the time to drop the ball when it comes to taking care of your mind, body, and spirit.

Hopefully, now that you're seeing just how possible it is to improve your overall health and reap the huge rewards that come with doing so, you're feeling a little better about being in this phase of your life but cast your mind back to when it all seemed a little more intimidating. This is your chance to reach out to other people who are feeling that way now and show them what they can do to take charge of their health.

The good news is that there's an easy way to do this, and it won't take more than a few minutes of your time. All you need to do is leave a short review.

By leaving a review of this book on Amazon, you'll show new readers the transformation that's possible when they lower inflammation, balance their hormones, and improve their gut health – and you'll show them exactly where they can find the roadmap that will get them there.

There are countless women looking for this advice, and at this transitional phase of life, they need the same reassurance and guidance that you're discovering here. Your review will help them to find it.

Thank you so much for your support. Life's too short not to live it fully.

ANTI-INFLAMMATORY DIET FOR WOMEN OVER 40

> "Your body hears everything your mind says. Stay positive, be kind to yourself, and watch your health flourish."
>
> — UNKNOWN

5.1: KEY FOODS THAT SUPPORT HORMONAL BALANCE AND REDUCE INFLAMMATION

A healthy diet is important to stay healthy overall, especially for women over 40. It can help regulate hormones and reduce inflammation. Since changes in hormones and inflammation can affect various aspects of health, including energy levels, happiness, and the risk of chronic diseases, it's important to know which foods can help balance hormones and lower inflammation.

Salmon, mackerel, and sardines are all fatty fish. These fish are high in omega-3 fatty acids, especially EPA and DHA, which are known to help reduce inflammation.

Omega-3s help lower inflammation by stopping the production of chemicals that cause inflammation. These fats also help maintain hormonal balance by keeping cell walls healthy, which is important for hormone receptors to work.

Chia Seeds and Flax Seeds:

- ALA, a plant-based omega-3 fatty acid, can be found in large amounts in both flaxseeds and chia seeds.
- ALA can help reduce inflammation and promote heart health. These seeds also have lignans, chemicals that may have estrogenic effects and could help women who have gone through menopause maintain their hormonal balance.

Berries (Strawberries, Raspberries, and Blueberries):

- Antioxidants like anthocyanins and quercetin are found in large amounts in berries. These help fight oxidative stress and inflammation.
- Antioxidants protect cells from damage and help with general health, such as keeping hormones in balance.
- Cruciferous veggies (Broccoli, Cauliflower, Brussels Sprouts): Glucosinolates are chemicals found in cruciferous veggies that help the liver in detoxification.
- A healthy liver is important for hormonal balance because it breaks down hormones and removes

excess estrogen.

- Leafy greens, like kale, spinach, and Swiss chard, are packed with minerals and vitamins, including magnesium and calcium. These nutrients help keep hormones in check and also help prevent swelling.

Spices Like Ginger and Turmeric:

- Curcumin, found in turmeric, is a powerful anti-inflammatory ingredient.
- Ginger contains gingerol, which can help reduce inflammation.
- Both of these spices can help reduce swelling and keep joints healthy.

Nuts and Seeds, Like Sunflower Seeds, Almonds, and Walnuts

- Nuts and seeds are good sources of fiber, vitamins, and healthy fats.
- They help maintain steady blood sugar levels and reduce inflammation. Their high nutrient content also supports reproductive health.

Avocado:

- It contains many polyunsaturated fats, which can help lower inflammation. It also provides essential minerals and vitamins, like potassium, which helps keep hormones and blood pressure in check.

Foods High in Probiotics, Like Yogurt, Kefir, and Sauerkraut:

- Probiotics are good for gut health and are linked to hormonal balance.
- Good gut bacteria can influence inflammation and hormone production, so consuming probiotics can help regulate the gut microbiota.

Lean Protein (Chicken, Turkey, Tofu):

- Protein is necessary for hormone production and cellular repair.
- Choosing lean protein sources can support muscle health and reduce inflammation.

Whole Grains (Oats, Quinoa, Brown Rice):

- Whole grains are good for you because they have fiber, vitamins, and minerals.
- They help keep blood sugar levels steady and lower inflammation since they have a low glycemic index.

Green Tea:

- Green tea contains catechins, antioxidants that reduce inflammation.
- It also helps you control your weight, which can have a positive impact on your hormone balance.

Bone Broth:

- Collagen and amino acids in bone broth help keep your gut healthy.
- A healthy gut can help your body absorb nutrients better and keep hormones in check.

Dark Chocolate, but Only in Small Amounts:

- High-cocoa dark chocolate contains flavonoids, which help reduce inflammation.
- Eating in moderation can be a tasty treat that might be good for you.

Adding these essential foods to your diet can help keep your hormones in order and lower inflammation. Eating various nutrient-dense foods and avoiding processed foods, sugary drinks, and fatty fats is important, as they can help cause inflammation and hormonal changes. Individuals may also have different food needs, so talking to a doctor or certified dietitian can help you get your hormones in order to achieve hormonal balance and optimal health.

5.2: COMPREHENSIVE NUTRITIONAL STRATEGIES TO COMBAT INFLAMMATION

To ensure one's overall health and well-being, it is essential to have a diverse selection of dietary programs that are effective in reducing inflammation. There is a growing awareness among individuals that chronic inflammation may be a contributing factor in the development of several diseases, including cardiovascular disease, diabetes, and autoimmune problems. For women over 40 facing specific health issues, planning their diet in a manner that reduces inflammation might be very beneficial.

To combat inflammation, the following is an in-depth look at how nutrition might be used:

Participate in a Diet That Reduces Inflammation:

Consuming a diet high in whole, unprocessed foods and including very few or no prepared or fatty meals. This approach is known as an anti-inflammatory diet.

Your diet should include a wide variety of whole grains, fruits, vegetables, lean meats, and healthy fats.

You Should Prioritize Omega-3 Fatty Acids:

- Flaxseeds, chia seeds, sardines, and fatty fish such as salmon, mackerel, and sardines are all excellent sources of omega-3 fatty acids, known to be effective pain relievers.
- Try to consume these foods regularly to reduce inflammation.
- Increase your consumption of foods rich in antioxidants. Oxidative stress is one of the primary contributors to inflammation, which antioxidants combat.
- Consume extra antioxidants by eating almonds, leafy greens, berries, and colorful vegetables.

It would help to go for healthy fats, such as monounsaturated and polyunsaturated, rather than saturated and trans fats. These fatty acids are found in olive oil, bananas, and nuts, among other foods. These fatty acids have the potential to reduce inflammation and assist in maintaining a healthy heart.

Limit your consumption of processed carbohydrates as much as possible. White bread, sweet snacks, and beverages with added sugar are examples of these foods. Consuming these can lead to more severe inflammation and an increase in blood sugar.

To maintain stable blood sugar levels, choose whole carbohydrates instead of refined ones, such as brown rice, quinoa, and oats.

To this, add ginger and turmeric to your diet. Both gingerol and curcumin have been shown to decrease inflammation. When you use these spices in your cuisine or when you drink tea produced from them, you may reap the health advantages that they provide.

Consume Foods That Are Rich in Probiotics:

- Probiotics can help reduce inflammation by maintaining the health of your gut's bacteria.
- It is possible to find probiotics in foods such as yogurt, kefir, cabbage, and kimchi.
- Stay away from processed foods and those high in sugar. Consuming a large quantity of processed foods and sugar may lead to inflammation that lasts for a long time.

- Consume less prepared meals and items containing additional sugars, as well as products with added sugars, and make a habit of reading product labels.
- It is important to be aware of certain dietary sensitivities since some individuals may be hypersensitive to particular foods that induce inflammation.
- You can minimize inflammation by identifying foods and beverages that worsen the condition and removing them from your diet.

Be Sure to Stay Hydrated:

- Proper hydration is essential for your health and may help reduce inflammation.
- Drink plenty of water throughout the day to ensure that your body continues to function properly.
- Consider the possibility of using an anti-inflammatory pill. When you consult with a medical professional, you might be advised to take certain vitamins, such as fish oil or turmeric, to decrease inflammation further.

Practice Mindful Eating:

- Being conscious of the foods you consume may help reduce stress, which is associated with inflammation.
- Remember to listen to your body's cues about whether it is hungry or full and enjoy your food.
- Maintain a healthy weight, as excess body fat can lead to the production of inflammation-causing chemicals.

- Achieving and maintaining a healthy weight through balanced eating and regular exercise is important.

Be Sure to Keep an Eye on the Serving Sizes:

Consuming excessive food may cause inflammation and weight gain. Therefore, it is important to watch the quantity you consume.

Using herbs and spices can improve the flavor of your meal and decrease inflammation. Some herbs, such as basil, oregano, and rosemary, and spices, such as cinnamon, can provide these effects.

Make sure that your meals are well-balanced. Each meal should include protein, healthy fats, and carbohydrates that are high in fiber.

This stabilizes blood sugar levels and reduces inflammation.

By adhering to these comprehensive dietary strategies, you can improve your health and reduce inflammation in your body. It's important to remember that dietary needs vary from person to person. Creating an anti-inflammatory food plan tailored to your specific health objectives and requirements is possible by consulting with a physician or a professional dietitian. These modifications to your diet have the potential to enhance your health and reduce the likelihood of developing inflammation-related disorders. This makes them particularly crucial for women who are over the age of 40.

5.3: CREATING AND ADAPTING ANTI-INFLAMMATORY MEAL PLANS

Making and following anti-inflammatory meal plans is an important part of improving overall health and well-being, especially for people who want to fight chronic inflammation. When the body is hurt or infected, it naturally experiences inflammation. But when it lasts for a long time, it can lead to health problems like heart disease, diabetes, and autoimmune diseases. Making meal plans that focus on lowering inflammation can be a very helpful way to treat and avoid these conditions. This is especially important for women over 40, who may have health problems that come with getting older.

Here is a complete guide on how to make and include anti-inflammatory meal plans in your diet:

Start with Whole Foods:

- Your meal plans should be based on whole, fresh foods. These include fruits, veggies, whole grains, lean meats, and good fats.
- There are a lot of nutrients and vitamins in whole foods, which help fight inflammation.

Make Sure Your Meals Are Well-balanced:

- Every meal should have the right amount of protein, healthy fats, and carbs.
- A well-balanced meal helps to maintain steady blood sugar levels and reduce inflammation.

Get Omega-3 Fatty Acids:

- Fatty fish (salmon, mackerel) and foods like flaxseeds, chia seeds, and walnuts contain omega-3 fatty acids, which are very good at reducing inflammation. Make sure that these things are always part of your meal plans.

Eat Lots of Colorful Vegetables:

- Bell peppers, kale, spinach, and carrots are high in vitamins and phytonutrients.
- Try to include a diverse array of colorful vegetables in your diet for their anti-inflammatory benefits.

Choose Lean Proteins:

- Lean protein sources like fish, tofu, chicken without the skin, and lentils.
- Proteins are essential for tissue repair and maintaining a robust immune system.

Choose Whole Grains Over Refined Ones:

- Use whole grains like brown rice, quinoa, and whole wheat pasta over processed ones.
- Whole grains have more fiber and nutrients, which can help lower inflammation.

Use Herbs and Spices:

Herbs like oregano, basil, and rosemary, as well as spices like turmeric and ginger, can improve the taste of food and help reduce inflammation.

- Try using different herbs and spices to make your food taste better.

Add Healthy Fats to Your Meals

- Add healthy fats like olive oil, eggs, and nuts to your meal plans. These foods contain monounsaturated and polyunsaturated fats, which can help reduce inflammation.

Keep an Eye on Portion Sizes:

- Watch your portion sizes to avoid eating too much, which can lead to weight gain and inflammation.
- When your body gives you cues when it's hungry or full, listen to them.

Stay Hydrated:

- Staying hydrated is important for your health and can help with inflammation.
- Drink plenty of water throughout the day to keep your body functioning well.

Plan Your Snacks:

- Pick healthy snacks like a handful of nuts, Greek yogurt with berries, or carrot sticks with hummus.
- Snacking on healthy foods can help you keep your energy up and prevent overeating during meals.

Think About Food Sensitivities:

- Some people may have certain food reactions that cause inflammation.
- To lower inflammation, find things that might be triggers and take them out of your meal plans.

Food Prep and Batch Cooking:

- If you want to make it easy to follow your anti-inflammatory food plans, you should try meal prep and batch cooking.
- Preparing meals and fixings in advance can save time and ensure that healthy options are available even on busy days.

Get Help From a Professional:

- Talk to a trained dietitian or nutritionist if you have specific food needs or health issues.
- They can give you unique advice and meal plans that are made to fit your specific needs.

Be Open to Change and Enjoy Variety:

- Be open to experimenting with new recipes and ingredients to keep your meal plans interesting.
- Including variety in your diet not only keeps meals interesting but also ensures that you receive a broader range of nutrients.

Pay Attention to Your Body:

- Notice how your body reacts to various foods.
- Adjust your meal plans and nutritional needs based on how your body feels about certain foods. Always prioritise what feels right for you.

Making and following anti-inflammatory meal plans is an active way to improve long-term health and reduce the chances of inflammation-related health issues. Always remember that everyone has different food needs, and what works for one person might not work for another. Because of this, it's important to ensure that your meal plans are tailored to your tastes, lifestyle, and any health issues you may have. Consistently keeping up with your anti-inflammatory meal plans can help your body fight chronic inflammation and help you feel better.

5.4: UNDERSTANDING FOOD SENSITIVITIES AND ALLERGIES

Food allergies and sensitivities are common health problems that significantly impact a person's health and way of life. This part will go into more detail about the differences between food sensitivities and allergies and what they mean for your health. It is very important to understand these problems fully because they are very important for encouraging healthy living, especially for women over 40.

What Are Food Allergies and Sensitivities?

People often use the terms "food sensitivities" and "food allergies" to refer to the same thing, but they mean two different immune reactions to different parts of food.

Food Sensitivities: People with food sensitivities, also known as food intolerances, have trouble digesting certain foods. Unlike allergies, food sensitivities do not involve the immune system's IgE antibodies. Instead, they are usually marked by stomach problems like bloating, gas, diarrhea, or pain in the abdomen. Common examples include lactose intolerance, gluten sensitivity, and fructose intolerance.

Food Allergies: Food allergies are immune system reactions that are set off by certain proteins in some foods. These reactions involve the release of IgE antibodies and can show up as a wide range of symptoms, from mild irritations like itching and hives to severe, life-threatening anaphylaxis. Some of the most common food allergies include reactions to peanuts, tree nuts, and shrimp.

How to Find Food Sensitivities

It can be hard to tell if someone has food sensitivity because their symptoms can be similar to those of other stomach problems. But there are a few ways to help find troublesome foods:

- **Food Log**: Keeping a detailed food log can help people track how their symptoms vary when they change what they eat. This can show trends and possible things that set off those patterns.
- **Elimination Diet**: With the help of a medical professional, people can go on an elimination diet to slowly cut out things that they think might be causing their symptoms and then slowly add them back in to see how they respond.
- **Tests for Diagnosis:** Some diagnostic tests, like lactose tolerance tests or blood tests that measure certain antibodies, can help identify food allergies. However, these tests might not always work, so it is important to seek a professional opinion.

Taking Care of Food Sensitivities

Once food allergies are known, they need to be managed by changing how you eat. Here are a few examples:

- **Intolerance to Lactose:** People who cannot tolerate lactose can choose dairy products without lactose or dairy replacements, like soy or almond milk.
- **Gluten sensitivity:** People sensitive to gluten can avoid foods made with wheat, barley, and rye.
- **Fructose intolerance:** People who are intolerant to fructose may feel better if they cut back on high-fructose foods and drinks.

Learning About Food Allergies

It's easier to spot food allergies because their symptoms are usually worse and happen right away. Some of the most common signs of a food allergy are hives, swollen lips or tongue, trouble breathing, and stomach problems. In the worst cases, food allergies can cause anaphylaxis, a life-threatening condition that requires immediate medical help.

Taking Care of Food Allergies

Avoiding allergens at all costs is the only way to manage food allergies. People who are allergic to foods must try to follow the following practices:

- **Carefully read the labels:** Food labels must be carefully read to find information about allergens. Companies that make goods must list any common hazards in them.
- **Inform Others**: People with food allergies should let businesses, friends, family, and workers know their dietary rules so they don't accidentally expose others.
- **Bring your medicines:** People with severe allergies often take EpiPens or other epinephrine auto-injectors to treat anaphylaxis responses.

What It Means for a Holistic Health Approach

For a comprehensive outlook on health, you must understand food allergens and sensitivities. These conditions can significantly impact mental and physical well-being. Recognizing and caring for them properly can lower inflammation, reduce stomach pain, and have possible long-term health effects.

People who are sensitive to or allergic to foods need to get help right away. This is especially important for women over 40 who may already be having problems with inflammation and changes in their hormones. Because these situations can worsen existing health problems, it is important to ensure that the foods you eat are right for your health.

To sum up, learning all about food allergies and sensitivities is important for encouraging healthy living, especially for women over 40. People can take charge of their health and well-being if they know the differences between these conditions, figure out what makes them worse, and use the right ways to control them.

5.5: RECIPES AND MEAL IDEAS FOR DAILY WELLNESS

What we eat every day is a big part of being healthy. Food directly affects our energy levels, mental health, and physical health. Here, we explore nutrition-dense foods and meal ideas that are good for your health everyday. By adding these innovative foods to your daily routine, you can start living a better, more fulfilling life.

Breakfast: A Good Way to Start the Day

There's a good reason breakfast is the day's most important meal. It gets your body going, gives you the nutrients you need, and sets the tone for the rest of the day.

Recipe: Health-Full Smoothie Bowl

A healthy smoothie bowl is a great way to start the day. Blend spinach, banana, Greek yogurt, and almond milk together. Now top the smoothie with fresh berries, chia seeds, and a drizzle of honey for added flavor and nutrition. This smoothie bowl is full of vitamins, minerals, fiber, and antioxidants.

- **Pros:** This food choice is not only tasty, but it also has a lot of vitamins and antioxidants that are good for your health and well-being.

Lunch: Getting Ready for the Afternoon

- Lunch is a chance to boost your mind and body, which will keep you going all day.

Recipe: Quinoa and Chickpea Salad

Put cooked rice, chickpeas, cucumber, cherry tomatoes, and fresh herbs in a bowl. Add a lemon vinegar sauce on top. This salad is full of fiber, plant protein, and important nutrients.

- **Pros:** The quinoa and beans provide extra protein, and the fresh veggies provide vitamins and water, keeping your energy and mind clear. And it tastes great!

Snacks: Mindful Eating That Fuels:

Eating healthy snacks can help you control your hunger, keep your blood sugar levels steady, and avoid eating too much at meals.

Recipe: Almond Butter and Banana Slices

Spread almond butter on banana slices and add a pinch of cinnamon. This breakfast is high in fiber, potassium, and good fats.

- **Pros:** Almond butter and bananas make a great snack for fighting afternoon tiredness because they are both high in heart-healthy fats and make you feel full.

Dinner: A Healthy Evening Meal:

For dinner, you can enjoy a well-balanced, filling meal that helps you rest and feel better.

Recipe: Baked Salmon with Quinoa and Steamed Vegetables

Marinate pieces of salmon in a mixture of olive oil, lemon juice, and garlic. Bake until tender. Serve with a side of quinoa and steamed broccoli, carrots, and asparagus to go with it. This meal is full of omega-3 fatty acids and fiber.

Benefits: Salmon's omega-3 fatty acids are good for your heart and reduce inflammation. Quinoa and vegetables provide a wide range of nutrients to help you sleep well.

Dessert: Pleasure Without Feeling Bad About It

Satisfying your sweet cravings can still be a healthy part of your diet.

Recipe: Dark Chocolate and Berry Parfait

Layer Greek yogurt with mixed berries and sprinkle dark chocolate chips on top. This dessert contains probiotics, vitamins, and a little sugar.

- **Pros:** Berries are a good source of vitamins and antioxidants, and Greek yogurt is good for your gut health. Dark chocolate is a tasty treat that can also improve your mood.

Staying Hydrated is the Key to Life:

People often forget the importance of staying hydrated, but it's essential for overall health.

Recipe: Infused Water With Fresh Mint And Cucumber

Adding fresh mint leaves and cucumber slices to a water pitcher. You will end up with a cool drink. This drink keeps you hydrated, helps your stomach, and keeps your face clear.

- **Pros:** Staying hydrated is important for brain health, physical ability, and overall health. Adding cucumber and mint to plain water enhances its flavour and makes it taste more delicious.

Making Plans and Preparing Meals is the Key to Staying Consistent:

It takes careful planning and preparation to make these healthy foods and meal ideas a part of your daily life. *Here are some tips to help you stay on track:*

- **Plan Ahead:** Make a list of all the meals you'll be eating this week, ensuring they include a mix of foods to keep your diet balanced.
- **Going grocery shopping:** Make a shopping list based on your meal plan to prevent impulse purchases of unhealthy foods.
- **Cooking in bulk:** Plan your meals ahead of time to save time on busy days. For ease of use, cook extra quantities and freeze them.
- **Control of Portions:** Be mindful of portion sizes to avoid overeating. Serving smaller portions can help you better understand the amount of food you consume.
- **Mindful Eating:** Take your time with each bite and pay attention to your body's cues for hunger and fullness.
- **Various:** Try new methods and types of food to keep your meals interesting and healthy.

In conclusion, include healthy foods and meal ideas.

Adding exercise to your daily routine is a great way to get healthy and stay fit. The meals we've talked about are delicious and nutritious, and they will help you stay healthy and boost your mind and energy levels. By making conscious choices and putting a balanced diet first, you can start a life-long fitness journey and look forward to a better and more energetic future. To live a good life, remember that what you eat is only one part of taking care of yourself. Don't forget to take care of your mental and emotional health, too.

EXERCISE AND MOVEMENT

> "*The more you eat whole foods in their natural state,
> the healthier you will be.*"

— *AMANDA KRAFT*

6.1: CUSTOMIZING EXERCISE PROGRAMS FOR WOMEN OVER 40

Regular exercise is an essential component of overall health and well-being, and it becomes even more important for women as they get older, particularly those over 40. However, exercise cannot be approached with a one-size-fits-all mindset. Developing personalized workout routines for women in this age group is essential to ensure that they obtain the most advantages while also considering their specific needs and expectations.

Having an Understanding of the Significance Concerning Customization:

As women age, they experience several changes, including shifts in hormone levels, decreased muscle mass, bone density loss, and changes in metabolism. These factors can influence their fitness goals and preferred exercise methods. Customization considers all of these adjustments, ensuring that training routines are safe, effective, and pleasant.

Evaluating the Necessities and Objectives of Individuals:

The first step in building a personalised fitness program for women over 40 is to evaluate their specific requirements and objectives. This evaluation considers various aspects, including the individual's fitness level, health issues, personal preferences, and particular goals, such as managing weight, improving cardiovascular health, or enhancing strength and flexibility.

Customizing Exercises for the Cardiovascular System:

Exercising your cardiovascular system is essential for maintaining a healthy heart, metabolism, and overall stamina. The process of customization involves picking cardiovascular exercises that are most appropriate for a person depending on their preferences and their current physical condition. Here are some options:

Low Impact Cardiovascular Exercises:

Physical activities that have a mild impact, such as brisk walking, cycling, or swimming, may be beneficial for women over the age of 40, as they minimize joint stress and reduce the likelihood of injury.

- **Interval Training:** High-intensity interval training, often known as HIIT, is a kind of exercise that can be adapted to the specific fitness levels of each person. It is known to be excellent for burning calories and improving cardiovascular health.
- **Dance and Aerobics:** Fun and engaging options, such as dance or aerobics classes, cater to individual interests while improving cardiovascular health.

Strength Training for the Maintenance of Bone Health:

Bone density normally decreases with age in women, which increases the likelihood of them developing osteoporosis. Strength training should be included in personalized exercise regimens to maintain bone health and support muscle maintenance. Some important factors to consider are:

Using weights, resistance bands, or workouts that require one's body weight can significantly enhance bone density and build muscle.

- **Focusing on Specific Muscle Groups:** Targeting areas like the legs, back, and core improves overall strength and stability.
- **"Progressive Overload"** guarantees ongoing muscular growth by gradually raising the intensity and resistance of the exercise.

Ability to Be Flexible and Mobile:

To prevent injuries and maximize day-to-day functioning, it is essential to maintain flexibility and mobility. Personalized fitness plans must include stretching and flexibility exercises customized to each person's needs. Practices like yoga or Pilates, which involve static stretching, may be included.

Core Strength and Balance:

For women over 40, exercises focusing on core strength and balance are particularly important. A strong core can improve posture, reduce the risk of falls, and support overall stability. Planks, stability ball work, and balance training drills are some of the workouts included in the customization process.

Listening to the Body:

An essential aspect of customization is paying attention to the body's signals. Women over 40 are encouraged to listen to their bodies and adjust their workout routines accordingly. Recognizing the indicators of weariness, muscular pain, or joint stiffness and changing routines as necessary are all part of this process.

Nutrition and Hydration:

Women over the age of 40 need to supplement their exercise routines with an appropriate diet and enough water. A key customization component is the provision of nutritional recommendations that are based on exercise goals, help maintain energy levels, and facilitate healing.

Consistency and Tracking Progress:

Personalized workout plans should emphasize the importance of consistency and progress monitoring. Regular evaluations are good for women over 40 because they help them stay motivated and adjust their routines to fit their ever-changing needs and goals.

Including Mindfulness and Stress Reduction:

Meditation and other forms of deep breathing exercises are examples of mindfulness practices that may be included in personalized fitness routines. They can help lower stress, enhance mental well-being, and strengthen the mind-body connection.

Establishing a Supportive Community:

Encouraging women over the age of 40 to participate in fitness programs or organizations specifically designed for their age group not only helps with motivation and accountability but also fosters a supportive environment.

Guidance from Qualified Professionals:

When it comes to tailoring workout routines for women over 40, expert help is often required. Certified personal trainers, physical therapists, and nutritionists are all professionals who may play an important part in developing and modifying individualized workout regimens.

Final Thoughts:

Customizing exercise programs to fit the unique needs of women over 40 is essential for their physical and emotional well-being and for ensuring long-term success. By adapting workouts to their specific goals, preferences, and physical conditions, women in this age group can enjoy the numerous benefits of exercise while minimizing the risk of injury or burnout. Customization allows women over 40 to embrace fitness as a part of their lives that is both sustainable and pleasant, leading to an improvement in their overall health and quality of life.

6.2: UNDERSTANDING THE ANTI-INFLAMMATORY BENEFITS OF REGULAR MOVEMENT

One of the key pillars of a healthy lifestyle is regular physical activity and exercise. Daily movement not only helps reduce inflammation but also helps in weight loss, enhances heart health and strengthens muscles—benefits that are widely known. Inflammation is a typical response to an injury or illness; nevertheless, it can become harmful and out of control if it is not adequately regulated. In this section, we will delve into the scientific rationale behind the effects of exercise on inflammation and why exercise is such an effective way of combating chronic inflammation.

Inflammation is a sword with two edges, just like any other.

The body initiates a complex biochemical process known as inflammation to defend itself. It is essential to have this ability to combat infections, heal wounds, and repair damaged cells. When it comes to inflammation, however, there are two distinct types: short-term and long-term.

- **Short Periods of Inflammation:** This immediate response to injury or infection is known as acute inflammation. It causes heat, edema, and increased blood flow to the injured area. Even though it only lasts briefly, acute inflammation is essential for the body to recover.
- **Extended Periods of Inflammation:** The duration of chronic inflammation is much longer than that of acute inflammation. It can occur gradually, often without any noticeable symptoms. Chronic

inflammation is linked to a variety of chronic diseases, including heart disease, diabetes, arthritis, and certain cancers.

The Importance of Chronic Inflammation in the Development of Disease

One characteristic shared by several chronic illnesses is inflammation, which persists over an extended period of time. This happens when the body's inflammatory response is continuously triggered, leading to low-level inflammation throughout the body. Long-term exposure to this condition may cause damage to cells and tissues over time, which can result in the development and worsening of a wide range of health concerns.

Poor diet, stress, smoking, and exposure to environmental pollutants are just a few of the factors that can contribute to chronic inflammation. All of these activities have the potential to make inflammation worse, yet regular exercise is a very effective way to decrease inflammation.

Inflammation may be reduced with the use of physical activity.

The relationship between physical activity and inflammation can be understood in various ways. As a result of your physical activity, your body goes through several changes that help regulate inflammatory processes:

- **Reduced Fat Tissue Accumulation**

Adipose tissue may contain a significant quantity of cytokines responsible for inflammation. Regular physical activity, which reduces body fat, prevents the production of these inflammatory substances.

- **Muscle Contraction and the Production of Cytokines That Reduce Inflammation**

Anti-inflammatory proteins, known as myokines, are produced when muscles contract in response to physical activity. When pro-inflammatory cytokines are present, these myokines operate in opposition to them, fostering an anti-inflammatory environment.

- **Increased Insulin Sensitivity**

Regular exercise makes the body more responsive to insulin, reducing the likelihood of insulin resistance and the inflammation associated with it, both of which are characteristics of type 2 diabetes disease.

A more effective defense against free radicals includes antioxidants, which fight free radicals and potentially harmful chemicals. The body produces more antioxidants as a result of physical activity. Free radicals have the potential to produce inflammation and reactive stress when there is an excessive amount of them.

- **Better for Gut Health**

Exercise is beneficial to the health of your gut because it encourages the growth of beneficial bacteria. Positive microorganisms in the stomach have been linked to reduced inflammation.

- **Reducing the Effects of Stress**

Getting some exercise is a fantastic way to reduce stress. The effects of chronic stress may make inflammation worse. This is why engaging in physical activity to relieve stress might indirectly help reduce inflammation.

The Importance of Various Forms of Physical Activity for Your Health

Various forms of physical activity have varying anti-inflammatory benefits, including the following:

- Aerobic exercise, which includes brisk walking, jogging, swimming, and cycling, is known to reduce the number of genes in the body responsible for inflammation. Aerobic exercise not only reduces inflammation but also enhances heart health.
- Many different methods of resistance training may help you create lean muscle mass. Some examples of this training include lifting weights, utilizing resistance bands, and exercising with your body weight. When you increase your muscle mass, your body becomes more adept at coping with inflammation.

- Yoga, tai chi, and other types of exercise help you become more flexible, balanced, and aware of your body. These benefits can be achieved through increased flexibility and awareness of your body. Because of the inflammation associated with these activities, the chance of being wounded may be reduced.

"Balancing" the Use of Exercise and Relaxation

Even though physical activity may be beneficial in reducing inflammation, it is essential to find a balance between physical activity and relaxation. Excessive training may exacerbate inflammation, increase the risk of accidents, and exhaust you. If you give your body sufficient time to rest and recuperate, it can repair and improve its ability to adapt to activity.

Remarks to Conclude

Understanding how regular movement can help lower inflammation is one of the most important things you can do to stay healthy and avoid long-term diseases linked to inflammation. Exercise, a natural anti-inflammatory medicine, helps decrease adipose tissue, increases the production of anti-inflammatory cytokines, improves insulin function, strengthens antioxidant defenses, and positively impacts gut health. There are several advantages to engaging in various forms of physical activity, demonstrating how essential it is to have a holistic approach to physical fitness. However, exercising smartly and finding the right balance between physical exertion and rest is key to maximizing the anti-inflammatory effects of exercise while simultaneously reducing the likelihood of overuse problems. By integrating regular physical activity into a healthy lifestyle and making it a fundamental part of daily routines, individuals can effectively combat chronic inflammation and improve their overall quality of life.

6.3: BALANCING CARDIO, STRENGTH, AND FLEXIBILITY TRAINING

A well-rounded exercise practice is important for good health and happiness. To do this, you need to find a balance between three important types of exercise: running, power training, and flexibility training. These things work together in different ways to improve health, prevent injury, and improve life overall. In this section, we will discuss how important it is to balance these factors and give some tips on how to make a complete exercise plan.

Heart and blood vessel health can be improved through cardiovascular training.

Workouts that raise your heart and breathing rates are called cardiovascular or aerobic workouts. They play a big role in improving heart health, which is important for overall health.

Here are a few important things to remember about the perks of cardio:

- **Heart Health:** The heart muscle gets stronger through cardiovascular workouts. This makes the heart better at pumping blood and getting oxygen to the body's cells. Heart illnesses like coronary

136 | THE ANTI-INFLAMMATORY BOOK FOR WOMEN OVER 40

artery disease are less likely to happen because of
this.

- **Taking care of your weight:** Regular cardio
workouts help burn calories, which makes them a
good way to control your weight and lose fat. It also
speeds up your metabolism, which can help you keep
your weight in check.
- **Taking care of your mood and stress:** Endorphins
are the body's natural mood boosters. They are
released when you do cardio. People who use them
say that they help with worry, anxiety, and sadness.
- **Better Lung Function:** Aerobic exercises make lungs
bigger and better at what they do, which means they
take in more oxygen and eliminate more carbon
dioxide. This improves lung health.
- **Endurance and stamina:** Regular exercise training
improves endurance and stamina, making daily tasks
easier and reducing fatigue.
- **Less chance of getting chronic diseases:** Heart-
healthy exercises help keep blood pressure in check,
lower LDL (bad) cholesterol levels, and decrease the
risk of developing type 2 diabetes and stroke.

The goal of strength training is to build lean muscle mass.

When you do strength training routines, your muscles are
tested against force. You can do this with tools, resistance
bands, free weights, or through bodyweight routines.

Because muscle training is good for you, here are some important points:

- **More muscle mass:** Strength training helps build lean muscle, enhance your appearance, and speed up your metabolism, making it easier to control your weight.
- **Bone Health:** Weight-bearing strength training builds bone health and lowers the chance of osteoporosis, a concern for many women over 40.
- **Avoiding accidents:** Strong muscles support joints better and lower the risk of injuries, especially in the back, knees, and hips.
- **Better Functional Abilities**: Strength training makes people stronger and more functional, which makes daily chores easier and lowers their risk of falling.
- **Body Fat:** Muscle tissue burns more calories than fat tissue when you're at rest. This explains why your metabolism speeds up as you do strength training and gain muscle.

Flexibility training can help you move more freely.

The goal of flexibility training, which includes things like yoga and stretching, is to make joints and muscles more mobile. Here's why stretch training is so important:

- **Injury Prevention:** Staying flexible lowers the chance of getting strained muscles, sprained ligaments, and joint injuries, especially as we age and naturally become less flexible.

- **Posture and Balance:** Flexible movements can help you stand up straighter and maintain your balance. It is very important to keep our backs healthy and stable as we age.
- **Reduced Muscle Tension:** Stretching activities help ease muscle tension and pain, which makes them especially helpful for people who don't move around much at work or in their free time.
- **Stress Relief:** Many stretching routines include deep breathing and relaxing methods to help lower stress and improve mental health.

Balancing the Three Parts

For a well-rounded exercise routine, you should plan to do all three types of physical training every week: strength training, flexibility training, and cardiovascular training.

Here are some tips on how to find the right balance:

- **Frequency:** Do a mix of aerobics, strength training, and stretching at least once a week. There could be three to five days of cardio, two to three days of strength training, and two to three days of flexibility training. It depends on your exercise goals and time constraints.
- **Variety:** Change your workouts within each category to keep things interesting and avoid hitting a rut. For cardiovascular exercise, you can run, ride a bike, swim, or dance. When you lift weights, you should work out different groups of muscles every day. As part of your flexibility training, try different types of yoga and stretching.

- **Progression:** Gradually increase the intensity and duration of your workouts to challenge your body and get fitter. For strength training, you might lift heavier weights, run farther for cardio, or do deeper stretches for flexibility training.
- **Recovery:** It is very important to get enough rest and heal. Make sure you rest days in between hard workouts and use healing methods like foam rolling and light stretching.
- **Consultation**: You should work with a fitness professional or personal trainer to make a fitness plan unique to your needs and goals.

To sum up, the key to a complete and well-rounded fitness plan is balancing physical, strength, and flexibility training. Each part has benefits that work together to improve heart health, build muscle and strength, make you more flexible, and lower your risk of injuries. By adding these things to your weekly routine and making your workouts fit your fitness level and goals, you can get all the health benefits of a well-balanced fitness routine.

Here is a table summarizing the critical points about balancing Cardiovascular Training, Strength Training, and Flexibility Training:

Component	Benefits	Key Considerations
Cardiovascular Training	• Improved heart health • Weight management • Mood and stress management • Enhanced lung function Increased endurance and stamina • Reduced risk of chronic diseases	• Frequency: 3-5 days/week • Variety: Try different activities • Progression: Gradually increase intensity • Adequate rest and recovery • Consultation with a fitness professional
Strength Training	• Increased muscle mass • Improved bone health • Injury prevention • Enhanced functional abilities • Metabolic health	• Frequency: 2-3 days/week • Target different muscle groups • Gradually increase weights • Rest and recovery are crucial • Consider working with a personal trainer
Flexibility Training	• Injury prevention • Improved posture and balance • Reduced muscle tension • Stress relief	• Frequency: 2-3 days/week • Explore different stretching routines • Deepen stretches progressively • Incorporate relaxation techniques • Rest and recovery are important

6.4: OVERCOMING BARRIERS TO REGULAR EXERCISE

To live a healthy life, you must work out regularly since it is good for your mind and body. But many people, especially women over 40, have issues that make it hard to work out regularly. In this section, we'll discuss some of the most common reasons why people don't exercise daily and give you some real-world ways to get around these problems. By facing these problems, women over 40 can begin an exercise plan that improves their health and quality of life.

- **Time Constraints:** Many people face this barrier because they have busy lives with work, family, and other responsibilities.
- **Action plan:** It's important to make exercise a goal. Start by adding your workouts to your daily schedule and giving them the same importance as your other meetings. Start with short workouts that get the job done and take up only a little of your time, like high-intensity interval training (HIIT). To be consistent, you should work out in the morning or during your lunch break.
- **Lack of Motivation:** This is a barrier because motivation can fade over time, making it difficult to stick to an exercise plan over time.
- **Action plan:** Set clear, achievable goals that align with your interests and lifestyle. When you're active, do things that make you happy, like climbing, dancing, or attending group exercise classes. Having someone hold you accountable helps you stay on

track, so think about working out with a friend or getting a personal trainer.

Physical Limitations:

- **Barrier:** Existing health issues or physical limitations can make it hard to exercise regularly.
- **Action plan:** Talk to a medical worker, like a doctor or nurse, to make a safe exercise plan that fits your needs and doesn't harm you. Low-impact activities like yoga, swimming, and riding can be great for people with joint pain or trouble moving around. Over time, slowly work on increasing strength and flexibility to overcome physical limitations.
- **Lack of Energy:** Feeling constantly tired or having low energy levels can stop people from being active.
- **Action plan:** For more energy, pay close attention to what you eat and how much sleep you get. Eat foods that give you lasting energy, like fruits, veggies, lean meats, and complex carbs. Getting enough sleep every night should be your priority. Start your workouts with less intense ones and build up to more intense ones as your energy improves.

Fear of Injury:

- **Barrier:** The fear of getting hurt while exercising can be a big reason people don't do it.
- **Action plan:** Lower your injury risk by warming up and stretching properly before and after each workout. Pay close attention to the right form and method while you work out to avoid injuries. As you

get stronger and more durable, slowly increase the pressure, weight, or resistance to lower your risk of getting hurt.

Accessibility to Facilities:

- **Barrier:** Limited access to clubs or other fitness facilities can make it harder to work out.
- **Action plan:** Explore home or outdoor workout options with little or no tools. Websites and exercise apps are just a few online tools offering guided workouts for people of all fitness levels. With these choices, you can work out whenever you want without going to a gym.

Weather and Seasonal Changes:

- **Barrier:** Bad weather can make it hard for outdoor workouts.
- **Action plan:** Think about ways to work out indoors when the weather is bad. Ensure you have the right workout clothes for each season so you can work out outside without any problems. When the weather isn't great, opt for doing something indoors instead, like dancing or indoor riding.
- **Psychological Barriers:** Low self-esteem and a poor view of oneself can make it harder to exercise.
- **Action plan:** Work on having a positive self-image and being kind to yourself. Pay attention to how exercise can help your mental health by lowering stress and making you feel better. To lower your stress and boost your self-esteem, make exercise

goals that you can reach. Using awareness and calming methods regularly can help you deal with stress and improve your mental health.

Lack of Social Support:

- **A barrier:** Insufficient help and guidance from family and friends can make it hard to maintain an exercise routine.
- **Action plan:** Tell people you care about your exercise goals and ask them to support and encourage you. You should join an exercise class or a group where you can meet other people who are also interested in health. A helpful group can make people much more motivated and committed by giving them a sense of belonging and holding them accountable.

Monotonous Workouts

- **Barrier:** Doing the same workouts repeatedly can make you bored with exercise.
- **Action plan:** Add different types of exercise to your fitness practice to keep it interesting and fresh. Try doing different physical tasks, going to different places to work out, or creating new workout challenges. Trying out different types of training can make your schedule more fun and help you stick with it.

In summary, women over 40 can get past common problems that keep them from exercising regularly by figuring out how to deal with them in real life. Focusing on exercise, setting clear goals, getting professional help if they can't do something on their own, and putting themselves first are all things that women can do to start a fitness journey that will improve their health and happiness. Don't forget that exercise is a key part of a healthy and happy life. You can get the benefits of regular exercise if you are determined and don't give up. Get over these things that are stopping you from exercising and live a happier life. In the long run, this will make your life better.

6.5: SUCCESS STORIES: FITNESS JOURNEYS OF WOMEN OVER 40

As you start your journey to get healthier, you'll come across many amazing success stories that show how strong, determined, and dedicated women over 40 can be. These stories, which are great for getting ideas, can teach you how these amazing people did what they did. In this section, we will learn about the amazing changes four women made in their lives through their fitness journeys. These stories show the importance of being consistent and patient, eating well, and caring for your overall health and fitness. They can inspire and help others on their journey to health and fitness.

Sarah's Journey to Fitness

About Sarah

Sarah, a mother of two who is 45 years old, had been struggling for a long time with being overweight and constantly tired.

Journey to Fitness

Before Sarah started her exercise journey, she knew how important it was to establish healthy eating habits. Her change started when she started going for daily walks. Over time, she added strength training and yoga to her routine.

What We've Done:

Over a year, Sarah's hard work and determination paid off. She lost 40 pounds, built lean muscle, and felt more energetic.

Important Point:

Sarah's story shows how important it is to take small steps toward exercise at first and build on them over time. For long-term success, her story shows how important it is to be stable and patient. Sarah's journey shows that long-lasting change is possible if you are determined and calm.

Maria's Health Improvement:

- **Background:** At age 50, Maria had a lot of health problems, such as high blood pressure and joint pain.
- **The journey:** Maria decided to put her health first by changing what she ate and adding different types of exercise, like swimming and riding.

- **What We've Done:** In six months, Maria's blood pressure went back to a healthy level, and her joint pain got better. She said that her general health, mental focus, and emotional health had all gotten better.
- **Important Point:**

It's clear from Maria's story that what you eat can completely change your life. It also stresses the importance of choosing workouts that are easy on the joints and don't put too much stress on them. The story of Maria shows how making small changes to your life can have a huge impact on your health.

Laura's Midlife Marathon:

- **Background:** Laura had never run before, but at 45, she decided to pursue an ambitious goal.
- **Journey to Fitness** Laura set her goal to finish a marathon and started her journey from not running to running a marathon. She started training with a "Couch to Marathon" plan and slowly raised the distance she ran.
- **What We've Done:** Laura reached her goal by finishing a run, which she had been working hard to do for months. Her story shows that even big exercise goals can be reached with constant hard work and drive.
- **The main point is that** Laura's story shows that anyone can reach their exercise goals, no matter how old they are or how much experience they have. It stresses the impact of consistent training, and unwavering commitment can change things.

Grace's Changes in Mind and Body:

- **Background:** Grace, who was 42 years old, was under a lot of stress and had mental health problems.
- **Journey to Fitness** Using mind-body methods as part of her daily routine, Grace put her mental and emotional health first. She liked doing things like light yoga, meditation, and being aware.
- **What We've Done:** Because of her hard work, Grace's stress levels decreased greatly, her mood improved, and she became more emotionally strong. Being able to think again improved her health and well-being.
- **Important Point:** Grace's story shows how important it is to take care of your physical and mental health when trying to get fit. It discusses how stress-reduction methods can change your health and how everything is connected to well-being.

In Conclusion:

These encouraging success stories of women over 40 show that there are many ways to improve your health and happiness through exercise. Even though each path is different, these stories all have things in common: how important it is to be consistent, how powerful a healthy diet can be, how important it is to set goals that you can reach, and how important it is to look at your physical and mental health as a whole. These stories show that everyone, no matter what age, can always reach their exercise goals. Women over 40 have shown that they can get healthier and fitter with dedication, hard work, and the right support system. For example, these stories show people that if they work hard and don't give up, amazing things can happen. They inspire other people to start living a better, more satisfying life.

STRESS MANAGEMENT

> "Wellness is the complete integration of body, mind, and spirit - the realization that everything we do, think, feel, and believe has an effect on our state of well-being."
>
> — GREG ANDERSON

7.1: THE DIRECT IMPACT OF STRESS ON HORMONAL AND INFLAMMATORY RESPONSES

Stress is a big part of our daily lives, and it has very bad effects on our health. While stress reactions in the short term are normal and help us adapt, stress that lasts for a long time can hurt our hormones and inflammatory systems. This chapter will discuss how stress directly affects hormones and inflammation, helping you understand the complex links between stress, hormones, and inflammation.

Hormones and the Stress Response:

In response to stress, our bodies initiate the "fight or flight" reaction, primarily involving the release of stress hormones cortisol and epinephrine from the adrenal glands. By speeding up the heart rate, improving attention, and using up energy stores, these hormones prepare the body to react quickly to a threat.

This reaction to short-term stress is necessary for life but becomes a problem when worry lasts for a long time. Chronic stress can lead to high levels of cortisol, throwing off the body's delicate chemical balance. This long-term rise in cortisol can hurt the body's chemical processes in several ways, including:

- **Impact on SEX HORMONES:** Stress that lasts for a long time can disrupt the production of sex hormones like testosterone and estrogen. In women, this disruption can cause irregular menstrual cycles, make it hard for them to get pregnant, and raise their risk of getting polycystic ovary syndrome (PCOS). It can cause men to have lower testosterone levels and have problems with their sexual health.
- **Thyroid Issues**: Stress can also affect the thyroid gland, which is very important for controlling metabolism. Long-term stress can throw off the balance of thyroid hormones, making conditions like hypothyroidism or hyperactivity worse.
- **Resistance to Insulin:** High cortisol levels can make insulin less effective, leading to insulin resistance and a higher chance of developing type 2 diabetes.

Stress and Inflammation:

Not only does long-term worry throw off the body's hormone balance, but it also affects how it reacts to inflammation. Inflammation is a normal part of the immune system that helps the body fight off injuries and infections. However, when it lasts for a long time, it's more likely that inflammation can lead to several diseases.

- **Dysregulation of the immune system:** Long-term stress can make it harder for the immune system to control inflammation properly. This can make you more likely to get illnesses and have autoimmune diseases, which happen when your immune system accidentally attacks your tissues.
- **More inflammatory markers**: Studies have shown that long-term stress can raise inflammation factors in the body, like C-reactive protein (CRP) and pro-inflammatory peptides. This low-grade inflammation that lasts for a long time is linked to many long-term diseases, such as heart disease, arthritis, and brain illnesses.
- **The "gut-brain axis"** lets the gut and the brain talk to each other in both directions. Long-term stress can mess up this axis, changing the gut flora and making the intestines more permeable. These changes can make digestive problems worse and systemic inflammation even worse.

The Dangerous Cycle

One very scary thing about the link between stress, hormones, and inflammation is that it could turn into a deadly loop. Stress can cause hormonal changes and long-term inflammation, which can then make stress reactions worse. For instance, changes in hormones can cause mood swings, worry, or sadness, and that can make stress levels even higher.

Taking Care of Stress for Healthy Hormones and Inflammation:

Knowing that stress directly affects hormones and inflammation makes managing stress even more important for staying healthy. Some ways to lessen the effects of stress are:

- **Techniques for Reducing Stress:** Mindfulness meditation, deep breathing routines, yoga, and gradual muscle relaxation are all stress-relieving activities that can help lower cortisol levels and keep hormones in balance.
- **Do some physical activity:** Regular exercise can lower stress and inflammation. Endorphins are natural chemicals that make you feel good, and exercise can help your body better control your hormones.
- **Healthy diet:** Eating foods high in vitamins, omega-3 fatty acids, and nutrients can help your body deal with stress and inflammation.
- **Getting enough sleep:** Good sleep is important for keeping hormones in check and dealing with stress.

Not getting enough sleep can worsen stress reactions and inflammation.

- **Social Support:** Strong social ties and help from family, friends, or support groups can lessen the effects of stress on hormones and inflammation.

In conclusion, long-term worry can directly affect the body's chemical and inflammation reactions, which can cause several health problems. Stress, hormones, and inflammation are all linked, which shows how important it is to take a holistic approach to health. People can improve their health and well-being by learning how to deal with stress and improving the balance of hormones and inflammation.

7.2: COMPREHENSIVE TECHNIQUES FOR EFFECTIVE STRESS REDUCTION

We all have to deal with daily stress because our lives are extremely busy and demanding. Long-term stress that isn't dealt with can severely impact our mental and physical health. To protect our health, we must use diverse methods to reduce and manage stress successfully. This section discusses several habits and methods that people can use daily to improve their stress management.

Meditation to Help You Be More Mindful:

Mindfulness meditation has been around for a long time and is known for its benefits to mental well-being and stress reduction. Mindfulness is mainly about being aware of your thoughts and feelings in the present moment without any judgment. Mindfulness training helps people become more aware of their inner experiences, which makes it easier to deal with stressful situations.

- **Pros:** Mindfulness meditation gives people the tools to notice and accept their thoughts and feelings, which helps them control their emotions and deal with stress better.

Exercises for Deep Breathing:

People who are constantly stressed tend to breathe quickly and shallowly. One easy and effective way to deal with worry is to practice deep breathing. Diaphragmatic breathing and the 4-7-8 method encourage you to take thoughtful breaths that can help you slow down your heart rate and ultimately ease your stress and anxiety.

- **Pros:** Deep breathing techniques help you calm down by slowing your nervous system and lowering the body's reactions to worry.

Relaxing Muscles One by One:

Progressive muscle relaxation is an organized practice in which groups of muscles are periodically tensed and then relaxed. This practice helps you recognize and release physical worry, which is good for your mind and body.

- **Pros:** Progressive muscle relaxation helps people become more conscious of their bodies' feelings, which makes it easier for them to identify and treat stress-related muscle tightness.

Tai Chi and Yoga:

Mind-body techniques like Yoga and Tai Chi use controlled poses, moves, and breathing to help you feel better. These exercises not only make you stronger and more flexible, but they also help you relax and feel less stressed. Regularly going to yoga or tai chi classes helps connect your mind and body and helps you deal with stress.

- **Pros:** By bringing the body and mind into balance, Tai Chi and Yoga help relieve muscle stress, promote rest, and boost general health.

Biofeedback:

Biofeedback is a type of therapy that tells people in real time about events in their bodies, like their skin temperature, heart rate, and muscle stress. By monitoring these physical processes, people can learn to manage how their bodies react to stress.

- **Pros:** Biofeedback gives people the tools they need to understand how worry affects their bodies, which helps them learn how to control their reactions.

Cognitive Behavioral Therapy (CBT):

Cognitive behavioral therapy (CBT) is an organized way to help people find and change the unhealthy ways of thinking and acting that cause stress and worry. People can learn better ways to deal with stress and problems through cognitive behavioral therapy (CBT).

- **Pros:** Cognitive behavioral therapy (CBT) teaches people to question and change bad thought habits, which helps them better deal with stress and be emotionally strong.

Managing Your Time and Setting Priorities:

Managing your time effectively is a key part of lowering the stress from work and other daily tasks. Learning to set attainable goals, plan tasks, and use time well can greatly reduce stress.

- **Benefits:** People who know how to manage their time can get more done and feel less stressed because they feel they're in control of their tasks.

Support and Connection with Others:

Building and maintaining strong social connections and a support system is key to lowering stress. Getting involved with support groups, friends, or family gives you important mental support and a sense of belonging.

- **Pros:** Social ties are very important for mental health because they allow people to talk about their problems and ask for help when things get tough.

Making Choices for a Healthy Lifestyle:

Adopting a healthy lifestyle is part of a holistic approach to dealing with stress. Eating a healthy diet, working out regularly, and getting enough sleep are all important for overall health. Endorphins are natural chemicals that improve happiness and reduce stress. They are released when you exercise.

- **Pros:** Living a healthy life strengthens your body and mind, making it easier to deal with worry.

Getting Help From a Professional:

When constant and overwhelming worry gets in the way of daily life, it may be time to get help from a doctor or psychologist. These experts can help with specific problems and give advice based on facts that meet each person's needs. Therapy is especially helpful for dealing with mental health problems caused by long-term stress and figuring out what stressed you out in the first place.

- **Pros:** People who get professional help can learn specific techniques and therapy treatments to deal with chronic stress.

In Conclusion:

To sum up, effective ways to lower stress include many actions and habits that deal with mental, emotional, and physical stress. By using these techniques every day, people can make themselves stronger, improve how they deal with stress, and improve their general quality of life. It is important to remember that different methods work for different people. This highlights the importance of trying different things to find the best ones. The end goal is to create a unique stress management kit that gives each person the tools to deal with life's difficulties more easily and with greater strength.

7.3: THE ROLE OF MINDFULNESS AND MEDITATION IN STRESS MANAGEMENT

Stress has become a regular part of many people's lives in this fast-paced and often busy time. People can feel mentally and physically worn out from the pressures of work, family, and daily tasks. Thankfully, there are effective ways to deal with stress and lower it. Mindfulness and meditation are two of the most well-known. In this section, we'll talk about how you can deal with stress better by being mindful and meditating. We will talk about how they work, what benefits they offer, and how you can use them in real life.

How to Understand Mindfulness:

With an open mind and no judgment, mindfulness is a mental state in which you are very aware of the present moment. It means consciously noticing your thoughts, feelings, and sensations as they arise without trying to change or push them away. Instead, learn to look at these things with interest and understanding.

Meditation as a Way to Practice Mindfulness:

Mindfulness can be developed in an organized way through meditation. It's about setting aside time and space to focus on breathing, body sensations, thoughts, or specific objects of meditation. There are many different ways to meditate, but they all have the same goal: to train the mind to be present and aware.

The Ways That Mindfulness and Meditation Work:

Mindfulness and meditation have more than one effect on stress:

- **Getting rid of stress:** The body's calm reaction is set off by mindfulness and meditation, which causes stress chemicals like cortisol levels to drop. Because of this change in the body, the person starts to feel calmer and less tense.
- **Controlling your emotions:** These activities make you smarter emotionally and better able to control your feelings. By being aware of your feelings without judging them, you can handle tough situations better, which lowers the mental burden of stress.
- **Better brain functions:** Mindfulness and meditation improve brain skills like remembering, attention, and decision-making. This way, people can better deal with pressure and find good answers.
- **Building resilience:** Regular practice improves the brain's ability to deal with stress and problems. It also helps the brain change, which lets people recover faster from stressful events.

Pros of Being Mindful and Meditation:

Making awareness and meditation a part of your daily life has many benefits, including:

- **Getting rid of stress:** One of the biggest and most obvious effects is that people feel less stressed. Many say that awareness or meditation makes them feel calmer and more in control.

- **More emotionally healthy:** Mindfulness techniques help you control your emotions, making it easier to deal with stress, sadness, and anger. They also improve your general mental health, making you happier and more satisfied with your life.
- **Better Focus:** Mindfulness and meditation can help you focus and pay attention better, which can be especially helpful for lowering stress from work or daily tasks.
- **Get a better night's sleep:** Many people have trouble sleeping because they are stressed. Meditation and mindfulness can help people calm their bodies and thoughts, leading to better sleep.
- **Increased Resilience:** Regular practice increases resilience, which makes it easier to get back on your feet after a failure or stressor.

Uses in Real Life:

Mindfulness and meditation can be easily incorporated into daily life and changed to fit different habits. *Here are some useful ways to put these techniques together:*

- **Breathing with awareness:** Focusing on your breath for a few minutes daily can help you become more aware. Please pay attention to your breath without trying to change it. When your mind slips, bring it back.

- **Meditations with a guide:** Many apps and tools offer guided meditation practices that offer organized practices for different goals, such as lowering stress, improving sleep, or balancing emotions.
- **Walking with awareness:** An easy and effective way to add awareness to your everyday life is to practice it while walking daily. Pay attention to how your body feels with each step.
- **Mindful Eating:** Eating can become mindful if you pay full attention to your food's tastes, textures, and smells.
- **Moments of Mindfulness:** Mindfulness can be used in everyday tasks like dishes, showering, or waiting in line. These little acts of being present can add up.

Finally, awareness and meditation are indeed powerful tools for managing and reducing stress. They are helpful for mental and emotional health because they make you more aware, help you control your feelings, and make your brain work better. People can change how they deal with stress by incorporating these practices into their daily lives. This can make them more resilient and happy with their lives in general. Remember that awareness and meditation, like any other skill, need time and practice to improve. The benefits become clearer over time, which makes these habits a good investment in your health and well-being.

Here is a table summarizing the key points about the Role of Mindfulness and Meditation in Stress Management:

Aspect	Description
Definition of Mindfulness	Mindfulness is a mental state characterized by heightened awareness of the present moment with a non-judgmental attitude.
Meditation as a Mindfulness Practice	Meditation is a structured approach to cultivating mindfulness, involving dedicated time to focus on specific aspects.
Mechanisms Behind Mindfulness and Meditation	Mindfulness and meditation impact stress through stress reduction, emotional regulation, improved cognitive function, and resilience building.
Benefits of Mindfulness and Meditation	Benefits include reduced stress levels, improved emotional well-being, enhanced concentration, better sleep, and increased resilience.
Practical Applications	Integrating mindfulness and meditation into daily life through mindful breathing, guided meditations, mindful walking, eating, and moments.

This table provides a concise overview of the role of mindfulness and meditation in stress management.

7.4: BALANCING WORK, LIFE, AND SELF-CARE

Especially for women over 40, finding a balance between work, home life, and self-care is crucial for overall health in today's fast-paced and demanding environment. At this point in life, there are often new problems to solve, such as health issues, family duties, and job tasks. Maintaining a balance among these aspects is important for your physical, mental, and social well-being.

Being able to balance your responsibilities can be hard.

Women in their 40s and older often have many different jobs and responsibilities. They may have hard jobs, care for kids or elderly parents, and do chores around the house. If they don't handle this juggling act well, it can cause long-term stress and burnout.

Why Taking Care of Yourself is Important:

Self-care is not just a nice activity. It's a must, especially for women over 40. Putting yourself first means understanding that your health is the most important thing. It means making time for things that are good for your physical, social, and emotional health. Some of these things include exercise, learning to rest, having hobbies, and spending time with people you care about.

Being Aware of Stress and Burnout:

Women in this age group worry about burnout and long-term stress. Feeling emotionally drained, performing poorly, and not caring about anything are all signs of burnout. Stress that lasts for a long time can cause many health problems, such as high blood pressure, sleeplessness, and a weaker immune system. The first thing that needs to be done to deal with stress and burnout is to recognize their signs.

How to Find a Balance Between Work and Life:

It takes conscious effort to find a balance between work and home life. Setting boundaries at work, delegating work to other people, and putting yourself first can all help with this. Managing your time and staying organized are very important skills for this task. It can also be easier to handle your tasks if you ask for help from family and coworkers.

Why Taking Care of Yourself Can Help You Deal With Stress:

One of the best ways to lower stress is to look after yourself. Endorphins are chemicals that make you feel good and lower your stress levels. For example, regular exercise produces endorphins. Meditation and deep breathing are two calming methods that can help calm the mind and lower stress. Hobbies and spending time in nature are also good ways to relieve stress.

Setting Up a Routine for Self-care:

It's important to create a self-care practice that fits your needs. This routine might include a mix of hobbies, physical exercises, and other ways to relax. Regularly planning self-care tasks and giving them the same value as other responsibilities is very important. A well-rounded self-care practice can strengthen you and improve your overall quality of life.

Support Systems and How to Get Help:

It's hard to balance work, life, and self-care; no one should do it alone. Having friends, family, and, if necessary, professional counsellors or therapists as part of your support system can be very helpful. It's not a sign of weakness to get help when you're feeling stressed or going through mental health problems.

Getting Used to Changes in Life:

When a woman is in her 40s or older, her life may have changed in many ways, such as her children moving out, retiring, or getting sick. Being able to adapt is a useful skill during these times of change. Accepting change and focusing on the chances it brings can help you grow and give you a new sense of purpose.

In Conclusion:

Finding a good balance between work, life, and self-care is a process that takes time and effort. This balance is very important for women over 40 to keep their bodies healthy, effectively deal with stress, and improve their overall health. Women can live full, resilient, and healthy lives by understanding their difficulties, putting themselves first, asking for help, and being open to change.

THE POWER OF SLEEP

> "*Good health is not something we can buy. However, it can be an extremely valuable savings account.*"
>
> — *ANNE WILSON SCHAEF*

8.1: THE CRUCIAL ROLE OF SLEEP IN WOMEN'S HEALTH POST-40

Restful sleep is an important part of staying healthy and happy, and it becomes even more important as people age, especially for women over 40. This chapter will talk about how important sleep is for women's health after age 40 and how getting enough good sleep can improve a woman's physical, mental, and social health during this phase of her life.

Balance of Hormones:

A big reason why sleep is so important for women over 40 is that it helps keep their hormones in order. During peri-menopause and menopause, women's hormones often change, with a decline in estrogen being the most common. Sleep disturbances, such as insomnia and poor sleep quality, can worsen these chemical changes. Getting enough sleep is important for keeping hormones stable, since this can help with menopause symptoms like night sweats, hot flashes, and mood swings.

Ability to Think and Reason:

Getting enough sleep is essential for maintaining cognitive functions such as memory, focus, and problem-solving abilities. As women get older, they may notice changes in cognitive performance. Getting enough sleep is one of the most important things they can do to stop this. Restorative sleep is important for brain health because it helps the brain store memories, process information quickly, and keep up with learning.

Emotional Well-Being:

Emotional health and sleep go hand in hand. Not getting enough sleep or getting bad sleep regularly can affect your mood and make you irritable, anxious, or depressed. Because of changes in hormones and lifestyle, women in their 40s and older are more likely to have these mental problems. By prioritizing sleep, women can better control their feelings, be more emotionally resilient, and keep a more positive view of life..

Taking Care of Your Weight:

As you get older, it can be harder to maintain a healthy weight. Sleep is very important for maintaining weight. Lack of sleep can disrupt the chemicals that control hunger, leading to increased hunger and, more likely, a desire for unhealthy, high-calorie foods. In turn, this can lead to weight gain and obesity, both of which raise the risk of many health problems. Getting enough sleep is important for weight management because it helps keep your body healthy and your hunger in check.

Immune Function:

Sleep is important for the immune system to work at its best. Our bodies naturally heal and grow new tissues while we sleep, and it also helps fight off infections. Not getting enough sleep weakens the immune system, which makes women more likely to get sick. For women over 40, whose immune systems may already be having trouble with normal aging, sleep becomes even more important for keeping their immune systems strong and their health in general.

Heart and Blood Vessel Health:

Women over 40 have a higher chance of getting heart illnesses. Sleep is very important for heart health because it lowers inflammation and checks blood pressure. Bad sleep habits, like chronic sleep loss or sleep apnea, can cause high blood pressure and a higher chance of heart disease. Getting enough deep sleep can help lower these risks and keep your heart healthy.

Health of the Bones:

As women age, they need to keep their bones healthy, especially during and after menopause, when bone mass tends to drop. Sleep is good for bone health because it helps the body heal and grow new cells. Women who regularly have trouble sleeping are more likely to get osteoporosis or break a bone. Putting sleep first can help bone structure and your body's overall joint health.

Final Thoughts:

Overall, sleep is very important for women over 40 because it affects their hormone balance, brain function, mental health, weight control, immune system health, heart health, and bone health. Women at this point in their lives need to understand how important sleep is and take steps to ensure restful sleep. By prioritizing sleep, women can improve their health, well-being, and quality of life as they deal with the unique challenges and chances of getting older.

8.2: HOW SLEEP QUALITY AFFECTS HORMONES AND INFLAMMATION

Sleep is a complicated and necessary biological process that affects our health, including hormone balance and inflammation. Understanding the complex link between hormones, inflammation, and sleep quality is very important for women over 40 who want to stay healthy. In this section, we will discuss how the quality of your sleep changes hormones and inflammation and why this is especially important for this group of people.

Keeping Hormones in Check:

Sleep is a very important part of controlling hormones. It affects the production and balance of Cortisol, melatonin, insulin, and sex hormones like estrogen and progesterone. Changes in sleep habits, like not getting enough sleep or getting poor quality sleep, can cause chemical changes.

Cortisol, sometimes called the "stress hormone," has a daily cycle, with the highest levels in the morning and the lowest at night. It would help to get enough sleep to keep this normal cortisol rhythm going. However, irregular sleep patterns or insufficient sleep can mess up cortisol production, causing stress levels to rise and even contributing to chronic inflammation.

- **Clonazol:** Melatonin, also called the "sleep hormone," controls the sleep-wake pattern. Because it is dark at night, the pineal gland makes it most of the time. Good sleep and a regular sleep plan help the body make enough melatonin, which helps you fall asleep and stay asleep. Melatonin is also an antioxidant, which means it also helps the body fight inflammation.
- **Insulin:** There is a strong link between sleep and insulin sensitivity. If you don't get enough sleep, your cells may become less sensitive to insulin, which can cause your blood sugar to rise and your risk of getting type 2 diabetes to increase. Since inflammation can be caused by high blood sugar, the quality of your sleep is very important for controlling inflammation through glucose control.

- **Hormones for sex:** Sleep can significantly impact the balance and release of sex hormones. For women over 40 who may be going through menopause and experiencing changes in their hormones, problems with sleep can make these changes worse. If you don't get enough good quality sleep, your periods may not come on time, your menopause symptoms may get worse, and your bone and heart health may be negatively affected.

Taking Care of Inflammation

Inflammation is a normal and important way for the immune system to deal with threats like infections and accidents. However, chronic inflammation, also known as low-grade or systemic inflammation, can harm your health and is linked to many age-related diseases, such as heart disease, diabetes, and some cancers.

- **Sleep and Pain or Swelling:** Sleeping is important for controlling inflammation. The body's repair and regeneration processes, including the immune system, happen during deep sleep. These healing processes can be slowed down by not getting enough or regular sleep, which can cause more inflammatory markers to build up in the blood. Lack of sleep over a long period of time can lead to low-grade inflammation that lasts for a long time. This can be bad for your health as a whole.

- **Markers of inflammation:** How well you sleep can change the amount of inflammation factors in the body. Some signs can go up when you don't get enough sleep. These include CRP, IL-6, and TNF-α. More inflammation and a higher chance of inflammatory diseases are linked to higher amounts of these markers.

The immune system's job is to: The immune system, which is a key part of inflammation, is closely linked to sleep. Sleep helps the immune system work better by increasing the production of immunity cells, antibodies, and cytokines, which control inflammation. Sleep problems can weaken the immune system, making the body more likely to get illnesses and possibly worsen chronic inflammation.

In Conclusion:

Finally, the quality of your sleep greatly affects hormonal balance and inflammation, which are both very important for women's health, especially those over 40. Putting good sleep habits first and doing things that help you sleep better can help balance hormones, lower inflammation, and lower your risk of developing age-related diseases. Women in this age group should know how important sleep is for their general health and wellness and take steps to ensure restful and healing sleep.

8.3: PRACTICAL TIPS FOR IMPROVING SLEEP HYGIENE

Good sleep is important for everyone's health and well-being, but it's especially important for women over 40, who might experience hormonal changes that make them more likely to have sleep problems. Sleep hygiene is a set of habits and behaviors that help you get a good night's sleep. In this section, we will discuss tips for better sleep habits to help women in this age group get better and how to effectively deal with hormonal changes and inflammation that might affect their sleep patterns.

Consistent Sleep Routine:

- To set a normal sleep routine, go to bed and wake up simultaneously every day, even on the weekends. Being consistent helps your body's internal clockwork work better and helps you sleep better.

Set Up a Relaxing Bedtime Routine:

- Create a routine before bed to tell your body it's time to relax. Reading, light stretching, or a warm bath are some examples.

Optimize Your Sleep Environment:

- Make sure your sleep environment is optimal. This means keeping the room at a comfortable temperature, blocking out light with blackout shades, and investing in good-quality, comfy couches and pillows.

Limit Screen Time Before Bed:

- The blue light from screens like phones, computers, and TVs can keep you from falling asleep. Try to turn off all electronics at least an hour before bedtime.

Watch what you eat and when you eat it.

- Eating big meals right before bed can make you uncomfortable and give you heartburn. Drink less alcohol and coffee, particularly in the evening.

Stay Active During the Day:

- Do regular physical activity, but limit your exercise right before bed. Working out can help you sleep better, but it should be done earlier in the day.

Dealing With Stress:

- To calm your mind before bedtime, try stress-relieving activities like progressive muscle relaxation, meditation, or deep breathing exercises.

Do Not Take Naps:

- Short power naps can be good for you, but long naps during the day can make falling asleep difficult at night. A 20- to 30-minute nap is enough if you need to.

Watch How Much Fluid You Drink:

- Drink less fluids before bed to lower the chance of waking up in the middle of the night to go to the bathroom.

Take Care of Sleep Disorders:

- If you have a sleep problem like sleep apnea or sleeplessness, you should get it checked out and treated by a professional. These diseases can have a big effect on how well you sleep.

Take Care of Hormonal Changes:

- Women going through hormonal changes, especially during menopause, should talk to a doctor. They can talk about possible hormonal treatments or other ways to deal with the sleep problems that come with hormonal changes.

Make Your Bedroom a Comfortable Place to Sleep:

- Spend money on a firm mattress and pillows that make you feel good. If noise is a problem, you might want to try white noise machines or earplugs. Make sure the room is cool and dark.

Don't Take Naps During the Day:

- Short power naps can be helpful, but long naps can make it hard to fall asleep at night. Take a short nap early in the day if you need to.

Stay Away From Alcohol and Coffee Before Bed:

- Both can make it hard to fall asleep. It's best to avoid these things in the hours leading up to bedtime.

Get Professional Help:

If you still have trouble sleeping even after trying to improve your sleep habits, you should talk to a sleep expert or doctor. They can identify and address your underlying sleep issues.

To sum up, women over 40 can improve the quality of their sleep and lessen the effects of hormonal changes and inflammation on their sleep habits by practicing better sleep hygiene. By using these tips and making their surroundings more sleep-friendly, people can get better, more restful sleep, thereby improving their overall health and reducing the risks associated with not getting enough sleep.

Here's a table summarizing practical tips for improving sleep hygiene:

Tip	Description
Consistent Sleep Schedule	Establish a regular sleep schedule by going to bed and waking up at the same time every day.
Create a Relaxing Bedtime Routine	Develop a calming pre-sleep routine to signal to your body that it's time to wind down.
Optimize Sleep Environment	Ensure your sleep environment is conducive to rest, including room temperature and bedding.
Limit Screen Time	Avoid exposure to screens (smartphones, tablets, and TVs) before bedtime due to blue light.
Be Mindful of Diet and Timing	Avoid heavy meals close to bedtime, and limit caffeine and alcohol intake in the evening.
Stay Active During the Day	Engage in regular physical activity, but avoid vigorous exercise close to bedtime.
Manage Stress	Practice stress-reduction techniques such as meditation and deep breathing.

Limit Naps	Limit daytime naps, keeping them brief (around 20-30 minutes).
Mind Your Fluid Intake	Minimize fluid intake close to bedtime to reduce nighttime waking for the restroom.
Address Sleep Disorders	If you suspect a sleep disorder, seek professional evaluation and treatment.
Manage Hormonal Changes	Consult with a healthcare provider to manage sleep disruptions associated with hormonal changes.
Create a Comfortable Sleeping Environment	Invest in a supportive mattress and pillows; create a dark and cool bedroom.
Limit Daytime Naps	Long daytime naps can disrupt nighttime sleep patterns.
Avoid Alcohol and Caffeine Before Bed	Avoid alcohol and caffeine in the hours leading up to bedtime.
Seek Professional Help	If sleep troubles persist, consult a sleep specialist or healthcare provider.

These tips are essential for creating an environment and routine that promotes better sleep quality and overall well-being.

8.4: THE CONNECTION BETWEEN SLEEP DISORDERS AND AGING

As you age, you experience different physical and mental changes, which are normal and unavoidable parts of life. An often-overlooked effect of aging that is often forgotten is how it affects your sleep. Sleep is important for your health and well-being as a whole. As people age, their sleep habits change, and sleep problems become more common. To help older people with their special sleep problems and improve their quality of life, it's important to understand the link between sleep issues and getting older.

Changes in the Way You Sleep as You Age:

As people get older, there are significant changes in sleeping patterns. A change in the circadian cycle, which is also known as the body's internal clock, is the most obvious one. Because of this change, older people go to bed and wake up earlier. Younger people are more likely to be "night owls," while older people are more likely to be "morning larks." These changes in the circadian rhythm can make it hard to sleep sometimes, especially if your social routine doesn't match these natural changes.

Loss of Deep Sleep (Slow-wave Sleep):

Deep sleep, also called slow-wave sleep (SWS), is very important for the healing of the body and mind. For some reason, getting older is linked to less SWS. This drop in deep sleep can make you feel like you're not getting enough rest, and you may feel tired and sleepy during the day.

Sleep That is More Broken Up:

Older adults often have more sleep in fragments, which means they wake up more often during the night. These awakenings can be caused by several things, such as pain, health problems, or the need to go to the bathroom. People who have trouble sleeping may not be able to get enough continuous, restful sleep.

More people have sleep disorders.

Sleep problems like sleeplessness, sleep apnea, restless legs syndrome, and random limb movement disorder are more likely to occur as people age. These conditions can make it hard for older people to maintain a good sleep schedule. Sleep apnea, in which breathing repeatedly stops and starts during sleep, is more common in older people and can make it hard to sleep and feel sleepy during the day.

Effects of Long-Term Illness and Medicines:

As people get older, they are more likely to have chronic health conditions, and many of these diseases can make it hard to sleep. Long-term pain, heart disease, diabetes, and nerve problems can all make it hard to sleep. Medications that treat these problems may also have side effects that make sleeping hard.

Stress and Psychological Factors:

As people age, they often have to deal with changes, such as retirement, losing loved ones, and health problems. Adapting to these changes can cause stress and worry, making falling asleep harder. Understanding how psychological factors can cause sleep problems in older people is essential.

Being Alone and Social Isolation:

Maintaining social connections, such as friendships and participating in activities, is important for mental and emotional health. However, older people may experience social separation and loneliness, which can make it hard to sleep. Being lonely and not spending time with others can make it harder to fall asleep and may lead to frequent awakenings during the night.

The Evolving Relationship with Health:

People with sleep problems are generally more likely to be sick. Medical illnesses that are already present can make it hard to sleep, and poor sleep can also worsen health problems. For instance, sleep apnea that isn't addressed can raise the chance of heart problems.

In conclusion, the link between sleep problems and getting older is complicated and has many sides. Sleep habits change with age, and the risk of sleep problems rises. However, other things, like long-term sickness, medicines, mental stress, and being alone a lot, also play a significant role. Realizing these problems is the first thing that needs to be done to fix them, help older people sleep better, and improve their overall health. Some ways to help this group of people sleep well include changing their lifestyle, getting medical help, and getting emotional support to lessen the effects of age-related sleep problems.

8.5: DEVELOPING A PERSONALIZED SLEEP
IMPROVEMENT PLAN

Getting enough good sleep is an integral part of staying healthy and happy. However, achieving healthy and healing sleep can be challenging for many people because many things, such as lifestyle, surroundings, and personal tastes, can cause problems with sleep. Making a custom sleep improvement plan is a smart and helpful way to deal with sleep issues and improve the quality of your sleep. In this section, we'll look at the most important steps and methods needed for making a personalized plan to get better sleep.

Evaluation of Current Sleep Patterns:

The first thing you should do to make a specific plan to improve your sleep is to look at how you normally sleep. This means keeping track of how long you sleep, how well you sleep, and any specific sleep problems you may have, like sleeplessness or sleep apnea. Keep a sleep log to track your sleep and find trends or causes that might make it hard for you to sleep.

Setting Sleep Goals:

To make a custom plan, you must be clear about your sleep goals. Think about what you want to get out of better sleep. Depending on your goals, you may want to sleep longer, wake up less at night, sleep better, or deal with a specific sleep problem. Having clear goals gives you motivation and helps your plan go correctly.

Changes to Your Lifestyle:

Many problems with sleep are caused by the way you live your life. If you want to get better sleep, you should make changes to your lifestyle that will help you sleep well. Some of these are:

- **Setting up a regular sleep schedule:** Your body's internal clock works better when you go to bed and wake up simultaneously every day.
- **Making a relaxing bedtime routine:** Doing relaxing things like reading or taking a warm bath before bed tells your body it's time to relax.
- **Getting the Best Sleep Environment:** Make your bedroom a good place to sleep by keeping it cool, dark, and quiet. You should buy a soft mattress and pillows.
- **How to Deal with Stress and Anxiety:** Anxiety and stress can make it hard to sleep. Integrating techniques for lowering stress, like deep breathing or meditation, can be helpful.

Food and Nutrition:

What you eat and drink can greatly affect how well you sleep. Please don't drink alcohol, smoke cigarettes, or use caffeine right before bed because they can keep you from falling asleep. Also, watch when you eat because eating heavy or hot foods right before bed can make you uncomfortable and give you indigestion.

Do Some Physical Activity:

Regular exercise can help you sleep better, but it's important to do it at the right time. It might be too exciting to do a lot of intense exercise right before bed, so it's better to work out earlier in the day. Aim for at least 30 minutes of mild exercise most days as part of your practice.

CBT-I stands for "cognitive behavioral therapy for insomnia."

Cognitive behavioral therapy (CBT-I) is a good way to treat sleeplessness. It's mostly about how changing sleep-related habits and thoughts can affect people. Working with a trained therapist can help you learn how to get better sleep, wake up less at night, and get over the worry of being unable to sleep.

Evaluation by a Doctor:

See a doctor if you have a sleep problem like sleep apnea or restless legs syndrome. A medical expert can give you a clear evaluation and suggestions for treating your condition. Continuous positive airway pressure (CPAP) devices, medicines, or other treatments may be used to treat the condition.

Taking Care of Medications:

Doctors may sometimes recommend sleep aids to help people with trouble sleeping. When taking these medications, it's important to follow the instructions and be under a doctor's close supervision because they could have unwanted side effects or interact poorly with other medications.

Monitoring and Making Changes:

It's important to keep track of your progress once you've started implementing your specific sleep improvement plan. Note any changes in the way you sleep and check to see if you are hitting your sleep goals. If necessary, be ready to adjust your plan based on what you see and the advice of healthcare professionals.

Being Consistent and Patient:

It might take time and effort to get better sleep. It is important to follow through with your plan and wait. You might not see changes in your sleep patterns and habits immediately, but if you stick to them, you can reach your goals.

Making a custom sleep improvement plan is a smart and effective way to deal with sleep problems and improve the quality of your sleep. You can greatly improve your sleep and general health by analyzing your sleep habits, making clear goals, changing your lifestyle, getting medical help when needed, and sticking to your plan. Remember that getting enough sleep is an important part of living a healthy life, and spending money on good sleep can positively affect your physical and mental health.

A Chance to Inspire!

As you feel your health and happiness improve, it's natural that you'll want to share what you've learned with others. Please do! This is information that all women over 40 deserve to know! You can help them find it now by leaving a short review.

Simply by sharing your honest opinion of this book and a little about your own experience, you'll inspire more women to take a holistic approach to taking care of their health and show them just how good they can feel when they do.

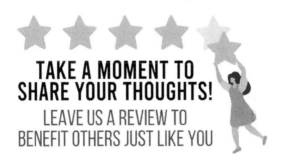

TAKE A MOMENT TO SHARE YOUR THOUGHTS!
LEAVE US A REVIEW TO BENEFIT OTHERS JUST LIKE YOU

Thank you so much for your support. Here's to a healthy and happy future!

CONCLUSION

We've covered lots of topics, strategies, and tips to help you take control of your health on this life-changing journey for women over 40. As this book comes to a close, let's review its main points again and send you a message of hope, support, strength, and a picture of your bright and healthy future.

Making a List of the Most Important Strategies and Techniques:

In these pages, we've discussed the most important parts of holistic health for women over 40. We've talked about inflammation, hormones, gut health, sleep, food, exercise, dealing with stress, and more. Thanks to these lessons, you now have a wide range of tools to improve your physical and mental health,

This is a Message of Hope and Empowerment:

Remember, your health is in your hands. No matter where you are in your health journey, you can make changes that matter. Accept the knowledge that comes with getting older and use that knowledge to push yourself to take care of yourself. Know that small changes add up to big ones and that your decision to live a healthy life is a powerful act of self-love.

The Road Ahead: Keeping Going on the Way to Health:

This book's ending isn't the end of your health journey. It's the beginning of a lifelong commitment to looking after yourself and living fully. Keep applying what you've learned and adjusting it to fit your changing needs. Accepting that happiness is an ongoing process and that every day brings new chances to grow and be healthy.

Support and Community Networks for Long-term Health:

Getting help and building a group around your health goals is a good idea. Talk about your struggles, victories, and life events with people who can relate and hold you accountable. Whether it's through support groups, family, friends, or online communities, remember, you're not alone in this health journey.

Last Thoughts: Looking Forward to a Bright and Healthy Future

Keep these last thoughts in mind as you start your next trip. Your health is a valuable treasure that needs your full attention and care. Accept that you are getting older with grace and confidence, knowing that each year gives you a chance to get stronger, smarter, and more alive. Take care of your body, mind, and spirit, and let your future show how amazing and full of life you can be by practicing holistic health.

Ultimately, this book has been your mentor, guide, and friend towards a happier, healthier life after 40. The information you've learned here is a present for yourself. It's a great trove of knowledge that you can use whenever you need help or ideas.

If you are determined, kind to yourself, and dedicated to your overall health, you are now ready to welcome a future full of energy, joy, and boundless health. Your journey goes on, filled with many paths to a brighter and healthier future.

Welcome it with open arms and a hopeful heart.

BONUS: BEST ANTI-INFLAMMATORY AND HEALTH SUPPLEMENTS FOR WOMEN OVER 40

Arnica: an age-old homeopathic solution, could potentially alleviate arthritis discomfort and soothe muscle pains.

Black seed oil: rich in antioxidants and bioactive elements, may promote skin and hair wellness, diminish inflammation, and aid in weight management.

Indian Costus: or Qust al Hindi, stands out as a highly esteemed herb with various advantages, such as aiding digestion, combating fever and infections, and potentially addressing severe conditions like Rheumatoid Arthritis.

Chlorella: aids in detoxification by assisting the body in processing heavy metals, combating the effects of processed foods, environmental pollutants, and other common stressors. Its ability to bind with heavy metals helps rid the body of toxins and supports hormonal balance by eliminating harmful substances found in food and the environment.

Zeolite: serves as nature's potent detoxifier, effectively eliminating free radicals and heavy metals. Crafted from a distinctive combination of volcanic minerals, it ensures optimal bioavailability. Enhancing brain function and promoting gut health are among its notable benefits.

Flaxseed oil: offers various benefits for women, including promoting smooth skin, strengthening bones, balancing hormones, preventing cancer, and more. Whether through supplements or including flaxseeds in meals, it's a valuable addition to maintain essential nutrients and a balanced diet.

Collagen: Research indicates that incorporating collagen supplements may assist in skin hydration and plumping, as well as improving bone density and increasing muscle mass.

Psyllium husk: a fiber supplement renowned for its capacity to alleviate constipation, reduce cholesterol levels, and maintain stable blood sugar.

Lecithin: Certain studies suggest that lecithin supplements could potentially lower cholesterol levels, decrease blood pressure, and alleviate symptoms associated with ulcerative colitis.

Turmeric: this golden spice, is thought to shield our cells from inflammation and damage, potentially slowing down the aging process, alleviating symptoms of arthritis, and possibly inhibiting the spread of cancerous cells.

Vitamin D3 and vitamin K2 work together to help your body absorb calcium effectively and direct it to your bones, while also preventing calcium buildup in your arteries.

Magnesium, along with vitamin B6, plays important roles in your body. It helps muscles and nerves work properly, regulates blood pressure, and supports a healthy immune system.

REFERENCES

- Chen, L., Deng, H., Cui, H., Fang, J., Zuo, Z., Deng, J., Li, Y., Wang, X., & Zhao, L. (2017). Inflammatory responses and inflammation-associated diseases in organs. *Oncotarget, 9*(6), 7204–7218. https://doi.org/10.18632/oncotarget.23208
- Furman, D., Campisi, J., Verdin, E., Carrera-Bastos, P., Targ, S., Franceschi, C., Ferrucci, L., Gilroy, D. W., Fasano, A., Miller, G. W., Miller, A. H., Mantovani, A., Weyand, C. M., Barzilai, N., Goronzy, J. J., Rando, T. A., Effros, R. B., Lucía, A., Kleinstreuer, N., & Slavich, G. M. (2019). Chronic inflammation in the etiology of disease across the lifespan. *Nature Medicine, 25*(12), 1822–1832. https://doi.org/10.1038/s41591-019-0675-0
- Admin. (2022, April 26). *How to navigate hormonal changes for women 40+.* Hormone Rebalance. https://www.hormonerebalance.com/how-to-navigate-hormonal-changes-for-women-40/
- World Health Organization: WHO. (2022, October 17). *Menopause.* https://www.who.int/news-room/fact-sheets/detail/menopause#:
- Gis. (2022, August 9). *Aging Digestive Tract - Gastrointestinal Society.* Gastrointestinal Society. https://badgut.org/information-centre/a-z-digestive-topics/aging-digestive-tract/
- Charlotte. (2020, December 16). How hormones affect energy levels. *BodyLogicMD.* https://www.bodylogicmd.com/blog/how-hormones-affect-energy-levels/
- Harvard Health. (2020, August 30). *9 tips to boost your energy — naturally.* https://www.health.harvard.edu/energy-and-fatigue/9-tips-to-boost-your-energy-naturally
- Spritzler, F. (2023, October 12). *What is an Anti-Inflammatory Diet and How to Follow it.* Healthline. https://www.healthline.com/nutrition/anti-inflammatory-diet-101
- Walder, C. (2021, September 24). *30+ healthy meal prep ideas for lunch & dinner.* Walder Wellness, RD | Simple, Healthy Whole

Food Recipes. https://www.walderwellness.com/healthy-meal-prep-ideas-for-lunch-and-dinner/

- Gazetteterrymurphy, & Gazetteterrymurphy. (2024, January 11). *Research shows working out gets inflammation-fighting T cells moving.* Harvard Gazette. https://news.harvard.edu/gazette/story/2023/11/new-study-explains-how-exercise-reduces-chronic-inflammation/

- *How to Reduce Stress through Mindfulness | Rehabilitation Research and Training Center on Aging With Physical Disabilities.* (n.d.). https://agerrtc.washington.edu/info/factsheets/mindfulness#:

- *Good sleep habits.* (2022, September 13). Centers for Disease Control and Prevention. https://www.cdc.gov/sleep/about_sleep/sleep_hygiene.html

- Chantelle. *40 Inspirational Quotes for Women in Their 40s.* I Am Brazen Spirit. n.d. https://iambrazenspirit.com/40-inspirational-quotes-for-women-in-their-40s/

Made in United States
Orlando, FL
12 September 2024